E. Landolt

Vade mecum of ophthalmological therapeutics

E. Landolt
Vade mecum of ophthalmological therapeutics
ISBN/EAN: 9783337815196

Printed in Europe, USA, Canada, Australia, Japan
Cover: Foto ©ninafisch / pixelio.de

More available books at **www.hansebooks.com**

VADE MECUM

OF

OPHTHALMOLOGICAL THERAPEUTICS

BY

DR. LANDOLT AND DR. GYGAX

PHILADELPHIA
J. B. LIPPINCOTT COMPANY
1898

INTRODUCTORY.

Our object in publishing this little work is to put into the hands of the profession a vade mecum containing in a concise form the indispensable facts of special therapeutics. This work is not a treatise of ophthalmological therapy, nor is it a dictionary, either of which would have made up a volume far larger than the small, easily portable guide, which we desired to produce.

It is our aim to give a constant companion, a true friend to the busy practitioner and to the student preparing for examination.

To facilitate the handling of our vade mecum we have arranged the headings in alphabetical order, thus saving the reader the trouble of looking up the index.

As the pharmaceutical part—the dosage of certain remedies and the most appropriate form of administering them—escapes the mind more easily than the general therapy, we have taken particular pains with our formulas.

It is clear that we could not enumerate all rem-

INTRODUCTORY

edies and formulas. We have limited ourselves to giving the most important, in order not to embarrass by the amount of matter those hurriedly looking up a subject.

Different type is used: for the general text; for titles at the top of the page; for the title of each article; for formulas, and for the method of their use.

Where method of application is not quoted under recipes it appears in the corresponding place of the text.

We have purposely omitted in our little work those modern forms of treatment, the therapeutic value of which is not yet established.

Nor did we describe the different operative methods, which would require a lengthy explanation or drawings or photographs. Our guide would in this manner have become much too voluminous to accompany the busy practitioner.

Our thanks are due to Professor Fournier, to whom we are indebted for the important chapter on the treatment of syphilis.

Mr. C. F. Haussmann, of St. Gall, the eminent chemist and pharmacologist, has had the kindness to review the chemical and pharmaceutical part of our little work. Without his help we would have committed only too many of those chemical heresies so frequently met with in medical literature.

INTRODUCTORY

The translation of the vade mecum into the English language has been made with the kind assistance of Dr. E. H. Neyman, of Milwaukee. We wish to express our thanks for the interest he has taken in the subject, and particularly for the considerable part of his time devoted to the work in question.

We must also not forget our publishers, who have acquitted themselves with as much good-will as success of their at no time easy task of giving this little volume the convenient form, which we hope will contribute to win for it a place, if not in the libraries, at least in the pockets of our colleagues.

OPHTHALMOLOGICAL THERAPEUTICS.

1. ACCOMMODATION, PARALYSIS AND PARESIS OF THE.

Search for and treat the *systemic disease*, cause of the paralysis [anæmia, disease of the brain or of the general nervous system, syphilis, diabetes, systemic poisoning].

Faradization: Positive pole upon the centre of the closed eye. Negative pole is passed along the orbital border, an even pressure being used.

Myotics [Eserine (111) or pilocarpine (251 a)]. —Paralysis of the accommodation being, as a rule, of long duration, limit the use of myotics to the time of eye work, and use strictly but the dose necessary to get effect wanted. Should the patient not stand the drug well, or should drug show itself inefficacious, add to the accommodation by convex lenses, adapting the eye to the necessary distance.

In cases of paralysis of *diphtheritic* origin: Strengthening food, open air, quinine (259), iron (164), hot baths.—Injections of strychnine (300 a).

In *rheumatic* paralysis: Ergot (109), salicylate of sodium (275), ointment of veratrine (318), of strychnine (300 b), or periocular massage.

2. ACCOMMODATION, SPASM OF THE.

Mydriatics [Atropine (23 a) or scopolamine (284)].—Rest; smoked glasses. Where there is hyperæsthesia of the retina, stay in darkened room.

As soon as the spasm seems fully overcome, lessen the dose of the mydriatic; work to be resumed gradually and carefully, beginning with *convex lenses* to entirely free the accommodation. Slowly the strength of these glasses can be diminished.

Acetanilid. See ANTIFEBRIN (14).

Achromatopsis. See DALTONISM (94).

3. ÆSORCIN.

Same use as FLUORESCIN (117). A 10 to 20 per cent. solution will stain the corneal erosion red immediately upon instilling. The red stands out better than the green of fluorescin on the colored background of the iris and the black of the pupil.

4. ALBINISM.

Smoked glasses. Where the nystagmus which frequently accompanies it is not very pronounced, stenopæic glasses.

Albugo. See LEUCOMA OF THE CORNEA (87).

5. ALCOHOL, ABSOLUTE (TEST FOR PURITY OF).

Add a small crystal of sulphate of copper to the alcohol; pure alcohol will remain colorless.

Alkali, volatile. See AMMONIA (10).

Aldehyde, formic. See FORMALIN (119).

6. ALUM.

a. Alum . . . . 2|50   38 gr.
   Rose water . . . . 50|00   13ʒ
   Distilled water . . . . 150|00   5ʒ

b. Pencil of alum, crystal of pure alum, *for cauterizations of the conjunctiva.*

Amaurosis, cerebral. *See* AMBLYOPIA and CEREBRAL AMAUROSIS.

7. AMBLYOPIA AND AMAUROSIS, CEREBRAL.

Treat the systemic disease [uræmia, typhoid fever, scarlatina, epilepsy, loss of blood, intense pain, hysteria.]

In cases where the cause is unknown: Absolute rest, darkened room, injections of strychnine (300 a).—Suggestion.—Eye-douches (99).

8. AMBLYOPIA, CONGENITAL.—AMBLYOPIA FROM LACK OF USE.

Where there is congenital cataract: Operate. —Iridectomy in case of corneal opacities.—Correct strabismus.

Methodical visual exercise of the amblyopic eye by itself several times daily five to ten minutes at a time. Correct astigmatism and aid accommodation according to needs with convex lenses.

Exercise eccentric vision. Where possible: Stereoscopic exercise to achieve binocular vision.

9. AMBLYOPIA, TOXIC.

Treat according to cause.—Stop tobacco and alcohol.—Milk diet.—Treat inflammation of stomach, digestive troubles, and insomnia (140). Carlsbad salts, tonics, hygienic diet.—Hydrotherapy (98), Turkish baths.

10. AMMONIA.

a. Ammonia . . . . } āā 10|0   2½ʒ
   Sulphuric ether or chloroform . . . .
   For insect-bites.

b. Carbonate of ammonia—"vola- } 0|50 to 2|0 8 gr. to ½ʒ
   tile salt" . . . .
   As a draught.

For instance :

Carbonate of ammonia . . . . 12|0   3ʒ
Distilled water . . . . 250|0   8ʒ
Syrup of althæa . . . . 50|0   1ʒ 5ʒ
   Tablespoonful every half-hour. In case of poisoning.

11. AMYL NITRITE.

Three to eight drops inhaled.

Anæsthesia. *See* CHLOROFORM ANÆSTHESIA (42) and ETHYL BROMIDE (113).

12. ANISOMETROPIA.

It is *impossible to give absolute rules* for the correction of anisometropia. One patient will be comfortable, refraction of both eyes having been completely equalized ; another will stand only a partial correction ; still another will refuse all glasses capable of lessening the difference in refraction between his two eyes.

Let yourself be led by the habit of the patient, and give preference to lenses that ease the effort at accommodation most if patient will not accept a full correction of his anisometropia.

13. ANKYLOBLEPHARON.

Surgical treatment.

Antidotes. *See* poisoning by ATROPINE (23), MORPHINE (231), PILOCARPINE (251).

14. ANTIFEBRIN, ACETANILID.

Antifebrin	0|25 to 0|40	4 gr. to 7 gr.
White sugar	0|30	5 gr.

One powder. *Take 3 to 5 powders a day.*

15. ANTIPYRIN.

a. Antipyrin . . . . 0|50 to 1|0   7½ gr. to 15 gr.

Powder every two hours. Not more than 5 to 6 powders a day.

b. Antipyrin	10|00	2⅓
Muriate of cocaine	0|15	2½ gr.
Distilled water	10|00	2⅓

For hypodermic injections: *One Pravaz syringe contains* 0|50 (7 1-2 gr) *antipyrin.*

16. ANTISEPSIS AND ASEPSIS.

a. Operating-room is aired and cleaned with greatest care.

b. Patient takes a complete bath on the evening before the operation. The whole head is washed with particular care. *For cataract operation:* Cut off lashes and eyebrows and brush the palpebral margin with sublimate solution 1 : 2000, or with biniodide of mercury (4 parts to 1000 parts of sterilized olive oil).—During the night, antiseptic dressing (101) of the eye to be operated. On day of operation, early, purgative; for instance, sufficient quantity Hunyadi Janos water (2 to 4 wineglasses). After movement: Opium (242 c), in order to prevent stools for several days.—An hour before soap, and sublimate solution 1 : 1000. Clean with operation the ocular region is cleansed with brush, the greatest care all the folds of the conjunctival sac with 1 : 5000 sublimate solution; thereupon aseptic dressing (sterilized cotton and bandage), which patient will wear up to the moment of operation.—*During operation* the field is washed when necessary with a physiological salt solution (6 to 7 : 1000) which has been previously boiled.

c. To disinfect the hands of *operator* and *assistants:* Wash with (1) Hot water, brush, potassium soap. (2) Alcohol. (3) Sublimate 1 : 500; dry with sterilized towel, or wear sterilized cotton gloves, which have to be removed when instruments are picked up.

d. Instruments are boiled in a physiological salt solution; they are not to be put into the solution before it has reached boiling point.—Less reliable proceeding: Instruments remain for 30 to 40 minutes in carbolic acid solution 5 : 100; oxycyanide of mercury 1 : 100, or solution of formaldehyde 1 : 500. Just before operation instruments are placed in sterilized water.—*Keep disinfected* needles in absolute alcohol (5).

e. Collyria are sterilized by boiling before each operation.

f. All *materials for dressings* (cotton, bandages, gauze, etc.) are subjected to the action of overheated steam (110° to 120° Centigrade) in a sterilizer during 30 minutes.

Antisyphilitic Treatment. *See* SPECIFIC TREATMENT (291).

Aphakia. *See* under the heading of HYPERMETROPIA (137).

17. AQUÆ AROMATICÆ.

[*Do not confound with aromatic spirits.*] Rose water, lavender water, fennel water, cherry-laurel water, aniseed water, balm mint water, thyme water.

In the treatment of conjunctivitis one can add these waters indiscriminately to the different collyria in the proportion of one-fifth.

In case of pain or itching, cherry-laurel water is to be preferred.

18. ARISTOL.

a. As a powder.
b. Aristol . . . . 3|0 to 10|0   45 gr. to 2½ʒ
   Vaseline . . . . 30|0   1ʒ
   Burns (of the lids); cover with gutta-percha.

c. Aristol . . . . 3|0   45 gr.
   Olive oil . . . . 20|0   5ʒ
   Lanolin . . . . 100|0   3ʒ 2ʒ
   Burns.

19. ARNICA.

a. Pure tincture of arnica.
   Rub into diseased parts.
b. Tincture of arnica . . . . 20|0   5ʒ
   Distilled water . . . . 150|0   5ʒ
   As compresses.

20. ARSENIC.

a. Fowler's Solution. (1 part arsenic acid, 1 part pure carbonate of potassium to 100 parts solution.)

Begin with 2 drops a day, gradually increase to 14, and decrease the dose again to 2 drops before ceasing.

b. Arsenate of sodium . . . . 0|003 $\frac{1}{20}$ gr.
Extract of gentian . . . . 0| 10 $1\frac{1}{2}$ gr.
Powder of gentian q. s.
To make 1 pill; 3 pills a day.

Asepsis. *See* ANTISEPSIS and ASEPSIS (16).

21. ASTHENOPIA, ACCOMMODATIVE.

Correct hypermetropia and astigmatism. Stop overwork and sexual excesses. Gymnastics. Sojourn in the country. Strengthening food, tonics. Hydrotherapy (98). Faradization. Compare also Paresis of Accommodation (1). For *muscular asthenopia*, see INSUFFICIENCY OF CONVERGENCE (142).

22. ASTIGMATISM.

a. **Regular Astigmatism**: After examination with ophthalmoscope or by skiascopy and with keratometer and repeated tests with glasses [if need be under atropine], correct the whole astigmatism with the corresponding cylindrical glass, adding, where necessary, a spherical lens according to rules mentioned. *See* MYOPIA (234) and HYPERMETROPIA (137).

b. **Irregular Astigmatism**: Correct as much as possible by spherical and cylindrical lenses that part of the ametropia which can be corrected. Stenopæic glasses.

Atrophy of the Eyeball. *See* PHTHISIS OF THE EYEBALL (250).

Atrophy of the Optic Nerve. *See* OPTIC NERVE (243).

23. ATROPINE.

a. Neutral sulphate of atropine . . . . 0|05   ⅚ gr.
   Distilled water . . . . 10|00   2⅔ℨ
   Instil several times daily; 1 drop each time.

b. Neutral sulphate of atropine . . . . 0|03   ½ gr.
   Muriate of cocaine . . . . 0|20   3 gr.
   Distilled water . . . . 5|00   1⅓ℨ
   Instil several times a day.

c. Neutral sulphate of atropine . . . . } āā   0|10 āā 1½ gr.
   Neutral sulphate of duboisine . . . .
   Muriate of cocaine . . . .   0|50   8 gr.
   Distilled water . . . .   15|00   4ℨ
   Instil several times a day.

d. Neutral sulphate of atropine . 0|03 to 0|10   ½ gr. to 1½ gr.
   White vaseline . . . . 15|00   4ℨ
   Put into conjunctival sac.

To get the *greatest possible effect:* Introduce the *pure salt* into the conjunctival sac, taking care to close the lachrymal ducts by pressure.

As a rule, let patient keep eyes closed for 5 minutes after having instilled the mydriatic.

In case of *poisoning by Atropine:*

a. Absorption *per os.*

Stomach-pump or hypodermic injections of a solution of hydrochlorate of apomorphine 2 : 1000 up to 30 centigrammes (5 grains).

b. Absorption *through the tissues* (injections).

Hypodermic injections of a solution of hydrochlorate of pilocarpine 5 : 100, repeated as often as necessary up to 60 centigrammes.

In *both* cases *internally:*

Brandy, strong coffee, carbonate of ammonia (10 *b*).

24. BALSAMUM TRANQUILLANS.

Oleum Hyoscyami Compositum.

Rub into skin of forehead and temples or on painful parts. Cover with cotton or oiled silk to prevent grease spots.

Basedow's Disease. *See* EXOPHTHALMIC GOITRE (129 *A*).

25. BATHS, MEDICINAL.

A bath should be from *200 to 300 quarts* for an adult; less for children.

There should be an *interval of at least 3 hours after a meal* before taking a bath.

Temperature of bath:

Cold bath 10–22	Centigrade.	(50– 71 F.)
Tepid bath 23–32	"	(73– 89 F.)
Hot bath 33–40	"	(91–104 F.)

a. Bran bath :

Add to the bath a decoction of 2–4 pounds of wheat bran.

b. Malt bath :

Pour 6 pounds of boiled malt through a sieve and add slowly to bath.

c. Salt bath :

Chloride of sodium, 8 pounds.

BATHS

d. Sea Salt bath :

Sea salt	} āā 4 pounds.
Chloride of magnesium	
Sulphate of sodium	
Chloride of lime	6 pounds.

e. Ferruginous bath :

e′. Sulphate of iron .... } āā 50|0   1ʒ 5ʒ
    Terra silicica ....
    Mix and dilute in water.

e″. Iron and potassium tartrate ...... } āā 100|0   3½ʒ
    Terra silicica ....
    As before.

f. Iodine bath :

Iodine	10|0	2½ʒ
Iodide of. potassium	20|0	5ʒ
Distilled water	250|0	8ʒ

Dissolve before adding to bath. Wooden *bath-tub*.

g. Sublimate bath :

Bichloride of mercury	25|0	6ʒ
Chloride of sodium	50|0	1ʒ 5ʒ
Distilled water	200|0	6½ʒ

Dissolve before adding to bath. Wooden *bath-tub*.

For the new-born reduce the dose of sublimate to 0|50; increase it to 1, 2, 3 grammes, etc., for older children.

Medicinal Foot-baths. *See* FOOT-BATHS (118).

Belladonna. *See* ATROPINE (23) and POULTICES (255).

Biborate of Soda. *See* BORAX (29).

Blennorrhœa. *See* BLENNORRHŒAL CONJUNCTIVITIS (69).

26. BLEPHARITIS, CILIARY, SQUAMOUS.—INFLAMMATION OF CILIARY MARGIN OF LID.

Minute cleanliness. Wash with soap and hot water. *Pluck out diseased lashes* (black roots).—Clean every morning from scales and pellicles with an ointment and a piece of soft linen [cold or tepid potato-starch poultices (255 *a*)]. Do not let the salve remain on lids too long; wipe off with care. *Never apply ointment just before retiring at night.*

Pay attention at the same time to any existing conjunctivitis. Watch the normal flow of tears through the natural passages, but avoid slitting the lachrymal ducts unnecessarily.

In case of *scrofula* and *anæmia:* Systemic treatment. Cod-liver oil (54), iron (164), sea bathing with certain restrictions (a well-protected beach without fine sand).

Mornings apply on the margin of the lids one of the following ointments, and let it remain there for one hour:

Yellow oxide of mercury (229 *a*), red oxide of mercury (229 *c*), iodoform (148), oxide of zinc (325 *b*), or, according to the case:

Salicylic acid	1|0	15 gr.
Oxide of zinc	10|0	2⅓
Powdered starch	15|0	4⅓
Vaseline	20|0	5⅓

Simple lead plaster	} āā 30|0	āā 1⅓
Linseed oil		
Balsam of Peru	1|0	15 gr.

BLEPHARITIS

Red precipitate of mercury	} āā 0	15 āā	2½ gr.
Camphor			
White vaseline	2 00		℥ß
Lanolin	1 00		15 gr.

Flowers of sulphur	3 0	45 gr.
Hydrochlorate of ammonia	1 0	15 gr.
Rose water	50 0	1 ℥ 5 ʒ
Spirits of camphor	10 0	2½ ʒ

Camphor	0 10	1½ gr.
Precipitated sulphur	1 00	15 gr.
Lime water	} āā 10 00	āā 2½ ʒ
Rose water		
Gum arabic	0 20	3 gr.

For *unyielding cases, apply this ointment* exceptionally every evening *to the border of the closed lids and let it remain until morning.*

White precipitate of mercury	0 03	½ gr.
Neutral acetate of lead	0 10	1½ gr.
Oil of sweet almond	0 50	8 gtt.
Vaseline	5 00	1⅓ ʒ

Red lead oxide	1 0	15 gr.
Neutral acetate of lead	3 0	45 gr.
Lard	45 0	1 ½ ℥

or:

White wax	} āā 20 0	āā 5 ʒ
Oil of sweet almond		
Oil of roses	3 drops.	3 gtt.

Against itching: Inunction, repeated several times a day, with resorcin ointment (260 *a*), or carbolic acid ointment (249 *a*), or brushing with:

Neutral acetate of lead	0 10	1½ gr.
Hydrochlorate of cocaine	0 15	2½ gr.
White vaseline	3 00	45 gr.

Blepharitis, Simple. *See* CILIARY BLEPHARITIS (26).

27. BLEPHARITIS, ULCEROUS.

In the beginning *always try the treatment of simple blepharitis* (26).

If there is no improvement: Compresses, with carbolic acid solution (1 : 100) to detach the crusts. Applications with a thin, pointed pencil of pure nitrate of silver, or with the mitigated pencil (287 *b, d*), or with a camel's-hair brush dipped in a 2 per cent. nitrate of silver solution. Wash the ciliary border of lids with glycerin soap, and make careful applications of 75 per cent. acetic acid to the ulcers; thereupon abundant bathing with hot water. *Careful* applications with oil of juniper (166 *b*), pure or with the addition of alcohol.

Where ulcers are *torpid :* Stimulate with tincture of iodine or with :

Crystallized acetate of zinc	0|40	6 gr.
Glycerin	5|00	1⅓
Cherry-laurel water	20|00	5⅓

In *unyielding* cases: Brush ulcers with a sublimated glycerin solution 1 : 30.

Repeat every other day.

Patient brushes border of lids *himself* with a solution of sublimate in glycerin 1 : 100, taking care that the solution does not get into the conjunctival sac. After the application: Calomel ointment (33 *b*) or :

Vaseline	} āā	5|0	1⅓
Lanolin			

Should *none* of these treatments *lead* to a *cure:* Cauterization with the galvano-cautery, or: Removal of the ulcerous part of the ciliary border.

28. BLEPHAROPHIMOSIS.
Canthoplasty.

Blepharospasm. *See* SPASM OF THE ORBICULAR MUSCLE (289).

Blue Stone, Blue Stick. *See* COPPER, SULPHATE OF (80 c).

Borate of Soda. *See* BORAX (29).

29. BORAX.—BORATE OF SODA.—BIBORATE OF SODA.

a. Biborate of soda . . . . 1|0 to 1|5   15 gr. to 23 gr
    Lavender water . . . . . . 30|0   1ʒ
    Distilled water . . . . 120|0   4ʒ

b. Borate of cocaine . . . . 2|0   ½ʒ
    Lavender water . . . . 50|0   1ʒ 5ʒ
    Distilled water . . . . 150|0   5ʒ

30. BORIC ACID.

a. Boric acid . . . . 20|0   5ʒ
    Distilled water . . . . 500|0   1 pt.

Calcined magnesia increases solubility of boric acid.

b. Boric acid . . . . 60|0   2ʒ
    Calcined magnesia . . . . 6|0   1½ʒ
    Distilled water . . . . 500|0   1 pt.

Boric acid solution, 12 per cent. (will not crystallize in the cold).

c. Boric acid, finely pulverized . . . . 25|0   6ʒ

In a large box; bring to each consultation for massage of the conjunctiva.

BROMIDES

d. Boric acid	0|25	4 gr.
White vaseline	5|00	1⅓ ℨ

Bran. *See* MEDICINAL BATHS (25) and POULTICES (255).

31. BROMIDES.

a. Bromide of potassium	10|0	2½ ℨ
Syrup of bitter orange-peel	30|0	1 ℨ
Distilled water	120|0	4 ℨ

Tablespoonful 2 to 4 times a day.

The bromide of potassium can be replaced by a little larger dose of bromide of sodium or a somewhat smaller dose of bromide of ammonium, or it can be combined with the two mentioned salts of bromine:

b. Bromide of potassium	3|50	55 gr.
Bromide of sodium	4|50	70 gr.
Bromide of ammonium	2|00	30 gr.
Distilled cherry-laurel water	15|00	4 ℨ
Simple syrup	25|00	6½ ℨ
Distilled water	110|00	3 ℨ 5 ℨ

Tablespoonful 2 to 3 times daily. (One tablespoonful contains 1|0 of the combined bromine salts.)

Where the patient does not stand the bromine well or where *prolonged use* is necessary, give after each dose a glass of carbonated water, or replace the above prescription by the following:

Bromide of potassium	1|50	24 gr.
Bromide of sodium	2|00	30 gr.
Bromide of ammonium	1|00	15 gr.
Carbonated water	1000|00	2 pts.

1 wineglassful 2 to 3 times a day. Avoid calomel applications while patient takes bromides internally!

Bromine. *See* BROMIDES (31).

Burns. *See* CONJUNCTIVA (57) and LIDS (192).

32. BUPHTHALMOS.

Try : Myotics, sclerotomy.—*Refrain from iridectomy.*—When troublesome : Enucleation.

Calcareous Infarcts and Concretions. *See* CONJUNCTIVA (61) and CORNEA (82).

33. CALOMEL. — MERCUROUS CHLORIDE.—MILD CHLORIDE OF MERCURY.

a. Calomel (by vaporization) . . . . 00|50   7½ gr.
   White vaseline . . . . 10|00   2⅓ ʒ

Introduce into conjunctival sac and make a massage of the cornea through the lid.

b. Calomel (by vaporization) . . . . 1|0   15 gr.
   White vaseline . . . . 10|0   2⅓ ʒ

Apply to border of lids.

c. Calomel (by vaporization) . . . . 6|0   1⅓ ʒ

In wide-mouthed bottle. Throw on conjunctiva and cornea with camel's-hair brush ; massage during one minute, wash with boric acid solution after 15 minutes to remove powder.

Once or twice daily.

d. Internally as a diuretic. . . . . . 0|05 to 0|1   1 gr. to 2 gr.

A powder.

Avoid applying calomel while patient takes iodine or bromine internally!

Carbolic Acid. *See* PHENOL (249).

Castor Oil. *See* OLEUM RICINI (274).

34. CATARACT.

Surgical treatment [see ANTISEPSIS AND ASEPSIS (16)].—Where not completely ripe or in case of zonular or punctated cataract, try to better vision by the use of mydriatics (233); instil scopolamin (284) in preference, as it can be used a long time without danger.

35. CHALAZION.

Always operate from the conjunctival side. Squeeze out the chalazion or excise on the finger-nail, using pressure of the fingers. [*Desmarres' forceps* is troublesome, painful, and *not necessary.*] Cavity should be scraped out with sharp spoon even where simple squeezing seems sufficient.

36. CHARCOAL, POWDERED.

Is *added* to *irritating salves.* The best is the charcoal prepared from the poplar-tree, as it releases the salts added to the ointment but slowly. It is sufficient to add 1 part of charcoal to 100 parts of the salve.

Preparation: Pound the charcoal in an iron mortar and pass through a silk sieve after having heated it to red heat during several minutes.

37. CHEMOSIS. — SUBCONJUNCTIVAL ŒDEMA.

Etiological treatment.—Ice-cold compresses.—Canthotomy.—Scarifications.

38. CHERRY-LAUREL WATER.

Is added to different collyria, particularly where there is pain and itching.

39. CHLORAL HYDRATE.

a. As a *sedative* . . . . . . 0|10 to 0|50   1½ gr. to 8 gr.
b. As a *narcotic* . . . . . . 2|00 to 3|00   30 gr. to 45 gr.
c. Chloral hydrate . . . . 5|0   75 gr.
   Syrup of orange peel . . . . 30|0   1ℨ
   Distilled water . . . . 60|0   2ℨ
   1 to 2 tablespoonfuls before going to bed.

To heighten the narcotic effect:

d. Chloral hydrate . . . . } āā 6|0   āā 1½ℨ
   Bromide of sodium . . . . }
   Syrup of codeine . . . . } āā 25|0   āā 6ℨ
   Cherry-laurel water . . . . }
   Distilled water . . . . 120|0   4ℨ
   1 to 2 tablespoonfuls before retiring.

Hypodermic injection:

e. Chloral hydrate . . . . 00|20   3 gr.
   Muriate of morphine . . . . 00|10   1½ gr.
   Distilled water . . . . 10|00   2⅔ℨ
   1 syringeful contains 0|02 (⅓ gr.) of chloral hydrate and 0|01 (⅙ gr.) of morphine.

40. CHLORATE OF POTASSIUM.

Chlorate of potassium . . . . 10|0   2⅔ℨ
Distilled water . . . . 300|0   10ℨ
Mouth wash; also brush teeth with solution during mercurial treatment.

41. CHLOROFORM.

a. Chloroform . . . . 40|0   1ℨ 2½ℨ
   White wax . . . . 10|0   2½ℨ
   Lard . . . . 90|0   3ℨ
   Inunctions against superficial extra-ocular pains.

b. Chloroform . . . . 20|0 to 30|0   5ℨ to 1ℨ
   Olive oil . . . . 40|0   1ℨ 2½ℨ
   Inunctions.

42. CHLOROFORM ANÆSTHESIA.

Pure chloroform poured on a sheet of white paper will produce the same sweet odor until totally evaporated, and leaves the paper absolutely dry, white, and odorless.

20 minutes *before narcosis:* Injection of 1 or 1½ syringefuls of:

Muriate of morphine	00|20	3 gr.
Neutral sulphate of atropine	00|02	⅓ gr.
Distilled water	20|00	5ℨ

1 syringeful contains 0|01 (⅙ gr.) of morphine and 0|001 ($\frac{1}{60}$ gr.) atropine.

5 minutes before narcosis: Apply a 5 per cent. cocaine solution to the mucous membrane of nose and pharynx.

For very anæmic individuals add several drops of amyl nitrate to the chloroform.

[10 drops to 50|0 (1ʒ 5ℨ) of chloroform.]

For patients with *heart trouble,* where narcosis is indispensable, replace chloroform by *ether;* give large doses of digitalis (96) several days before the operation, and let an injection of 0|001 ($\frac{1}{60}$ gr.) of strophanthin take the place of the morphine and atropine injection.

After narcosis cover face of patient for about 3 hours with a compress soaked in vinegar; renew it frequently.

Choroid, Detachment of the. *See* DETACHMENT OF THE RETINA (265).

Choroid, Hemorrhage of the. *See* HEMORRHAGE OF THE RETINA (266).

43. CHOROID, LESION OF THE.

Minute antisepsis; rest; ice.—Remove foreign bodies where indicated by means of the electro-magnet forceps, hook, or by aspiration.

Compare also PENETRATING WOUNDS OF THE SCLERA (282).

44. CHOROID, RUPTURE OF THE.

In fresh cases absolute rest.—Antiphlogistic measures.

45. CHOROID, TUBERCULI OF THE.

Enucleation in case diagnosis is absolutely positive.

46. CHOROID, TUMORS OF THE.

Tumors of the choroid are *all malignant*. Enucleation or exenteration of the orbit, according to extent of the tumor.

47. CHOROIDITIS, Plastic, Exudative, Disseminate, Areolar.—CHORIO-RETINITIS.—SCLERO-CHOROIDITIS.

In the *acute stage*: Leeches (186) to the temple and to the mastoid process, or Heurteloup's artificial leech (30|0 to 60|0 [1℥ to 2℥] of blood), or dry leeches, according to the patient's strength.—Absolute rest and darkness for 36 hours after bloodletting.—Derivation to skin and digestive tract.—Poultices (255); repeated hot compresses.—Mydriatics (233) as long as patient remains in darkened room; later, smoked glasses.

Methodical sweating (305); medicinal foot-baths (118).—Massage of the eyeball.—Repeated paracentesis of the anterior chamber.

When patient is *anæmic:* Strengthening diet. In case of *syphilis:* Specific treatment (291).

48. CHOROIDITIS, Suppurative, Metastatic, Purulent.

In the *beginning:* Compresses with iced water; mydriatics (233); antiphlogosis.

Where *suppuration* has begun: Hot compresses or poultices (255). Narcotics, and where the pain is great: Hypodermic injections of morphine (231 *c*) at temples.

No indigestible food.—Extraction of the swollen or dislocated lens.—Lengthy incision of the cornea or sclera to give vent to pus.—Exenteration (afterwards disinfection with sublimate solution 1 : 1000). Enucleation during remission of pain.

When suppurative choroiditis runs its course *without acute inflammatory symptoms*, as in young children, *special treatment is not required*. Simple hygienic rules generally suffice to hinder the suppuration from invading the whole eyeball.

49. CILIARY BODY, FOREIGN BODY OF THE.

Where extraction is impossible: Antiseptic (101) and antiphlogistic dressing and treatment. Should inflammation and symptoms of irritation of uveal tract increase: Enucleation or evisceration of the globe of the eye.

50. CILIARY BODY, MELANOSARCOMA OF THE.

Enucleation.

51. CITRIC ACID.

Citric acid	10|0	2½ʒ
Distilled water	150|0	5ʒ

52. COCAINE.

a. Muriate of cocaine	00|20	3 gr.
Distilled water	10|00	2½ʒ

Instillations.

b. Muriate of cocaine	00|20	3 gr.
White vaseline	10|00	2½ʒ

Introduce into conjunctival sac.

Hypodermic injections of cocaine may be used in lid operations, tenotomy, even in advancement of the muscles and enucleation.

c. Muriate of cocaine	00|40	6½ gr.
Distilled water	20|00	5ʒ

2 per cent. cocaine solution; 1 syringeful contains 0|02 (⅓ gr.) of cocaine.

d. Muriate of cocaine	0|80	12 gr.
Distilled water	20|00	5ʒ

4 per cent. cocaine solution; 1 syringeful contains 0|04 (⅔ gr.) of cocaine. 0|05 (⅚ gr.) of cocaine = maximal dose for injections in the periocular tissues.

53. CODEINE.

Phosphate of codeine	0|01 to 0|2	⅛ gr. to 3 gr.
Subnitrate of bismuth . . . . . . }	āā 0|50	āā 8 gr.
Sugar of milk		

1 powder every 3 hours.

54. COD-LIVER OIL.

In spoonfuls, large or small, according to age. Where there is fever and gastric trouble, cod-liver oil is not indicated.

The *light-yellow oil is the best,* extracted by an almost cold process, heat not having altered the active principles of the livers (iodine, chlorine, bromine, etc.), which are very volatile.—The light-brown oil is less active than the light-yellow, but is preferable to the dark-brown oil.

Should stomach revolt: Take often in small quantities, as:

a. Light-yellow cod-liver oil		1|0	15 gr.
In capsules—up to 15 daily.			

For children, use can be made of the aromatized cod-liver oil.

b. Cod-liver oil		500|0	1 pt.
Oil of cinnamon		15 drops	15 gtt.

For *scrofula*: Combine the cod-liver oil with extract of *malt* and *iodide of iron*.

c. Extract of malt		1000|00	2 pts.
Cod-liver oil		500|00	1 pt.
Gum arabic		100|00	3ʒ 2ɜ
Powdered tragacanth		5|00	1½ɜ
Glycerin		50|00	1ʒ 5ɜ
Vanillin		00|50	8 gr.
Iodide of iron		15|00	4ɜ
1 to 2 teaspoonfuls a day.			

55. COLLYRIUM, YELLOW ASTRINGENT.

Chlorate of ammonium		00|50	8 gr.
Sulphate of zinc		1|25	19 gr.
Distilled water		200|00	6½ℨ
Camphor		00|40	6 gr.
70 per cent. alcohol		20|00	5ℨ
Crocus		00|10	1½ gr.

Macerate 24 hours and filter.

Compresses of Subacetate of Lead. *See* LEAD (185 *c*).

56. CONIUM.

Powdered conium leaves		20|0	5ℨ
Lard		50|0	1ℨ 5ℨ

Heat on water-bath for at least half an hour; rub on skin of forehead and temples; acute pains of iritis.

See also POULTICES (255 *e, f*).

57. CONJUNCTIVA, BURNS OF THE.

Quick elimination of the caustic agents. In case of *burns with chemicals*, wash with

a. Oil or milk (quicklime).

b. Acidulated water (caustic bases).
   Teaspoonful of vinegar to a glass of water.

c. Lime water, or bicarbonate of sodium or of potassium (acids).
   Teaspoonful in a glass of water.

Remove scabs. Apply lukewarm 3 per cent. boric acid compresses.

To *avoid formation of adhesions:* Instil 2 to 4 drops of sterilized oil into the conjunctival sac until complete cure is effected, and pass a probe between the lids and the globe of the eye every day.—Later: Calomel ointment (33 a) or boric acid ointment (30 d).

58. CONJUNCTIVA, CYSTICERCUS OF THE.

Extraction after incision of the mucous membrane covering the parasite.

59. CONJUNCTIVA, HEMORRHAGE OF THE. — SUBCONJUNCTIVAL ECCHYMOSIS.

Compression.—Compresses with subacetate of lead solution.

Avoid straining, coughing, vomiting, etc.

In old people, inform family of a possible cerebral apoplexy.

60. CONJUNCTIVA, HYPERÆMIA OF THE.

Treat as chronic conjunctivitis (70).

61. CONJUNCTIVA, LITHIASIS OF THE. —CALCAREOUS INFARCTION OF MEIBOM'S GLANDS.

Incision of the mucous membrane following the course of the gland; remove the concretions with a small curette or knife.

62. CONJUNCTIVA, LUPUS OF THE.

General tonic treatment [iron (164), arsenic (20)].
Applications of tincture of iodine with a camel's-

hair brush or small pledget of cotton.—Excision of diseased parts. Scrape with sharp spoon.—Thermo-cautery.

63. CONJUNCTIVA, TRAUMATISM OF THE.

Remove foreign bodies.—Sew very carefully.—Antiseptic bandage (101) to be worn several days.

64. CONJUNCTIVA, TUBERCULOSIS OF THE.

According to extent: Excision or cauterization. Symptomatic treatment.

65. CONJUNCTIVA, BENIGNANT TUMORS OF THE.

[Fibromata, Lipomata, Cysts, Dermoid Tumors, Erectile Tumors.]

Excision; sew, having care to sacrifice the mucous membrane only as far as is strictly necessary.

66. CONJUNCTIVA, MALIGNANT TUMORS OF THE.

[Epithelioma, Sarcoma, Lepra.]

Where tumor is not too large and where conjunctiva alone is involved: Remove it. As a rule, a plastic operation will be necessary to avoid symblepharon.

Where the eyeball is involved, enucleation or exenteration may be indicated.

67. CONJUNCTIVA, XEROSIS OF THE.

Better the state of the general health. Wash frequently with biborate of soda (29). Instil milk or fresh oil.

68. CONJUNCTIVITIS.

General rules: Use *lukewarm* collyria. Do *not* content yourself with *simple instillations*, but *turn the lids* and *brush them.*—Between treatments patient is told to wash out and bathe his eyes, using absorbent cotton and an eye-cup.—*Dry eyes after applications, and avoid going out immediately afterwards.*

One can add to the collyria diverse *aqueous* (never alcoholic) aromatic solutions. Cherry-laurel water seems to be slightly soothing.

69. CONJUNCTIVITIS, BLENNORRHŒAL.—OPHTHALMIA OF THE NEW-BORN.

Prophylaxis: Where we find a suspicious white flow: Antiseptic vaginal injections before confinement.—In all children (mother having white flow), without exception, immediately after birth and before bath: Abundant washing of the lids and the surroundings of the eye with a 1:2000 sublimate solution and instillation of one drop of a nitrate of silver solution (2 per cent.).

Where one eye alone is infected protect the other by a watch-glass hermetically laid on, or, better, by an antiseptic dressing, covered by a layer of collo-

CONJUNCTIVITIS

dion adhering to the skin.—Tie the hands of the new-born.

Inform the mother, nurses, and all persons that come near the child of the danger of contagion.— Have the linen of the child carefully laid aside, as well as all dressings. Burn cotton used for washing the eyes. Wash your hands after each dressing with soap, brush, and sublimate 1 : 1000.

As long as the swelling lasts: Iced sublimate compresses (1 : 5000); remove every trace of pus carefully and regularly. To avoid borders of lids getting glued together, put between them a little vaseline ointment, with peroxide of hydrogen (135 *b*), or some of the following ointment:

White wax	3|0	45 gr.
Spermaceti	2|0	30 gr.
Oil of sweet almond	15|0	43

If necessary: Scarifications, followed by energetic sublimate washes (1 : 500).—Blepharorrhaphy.—Leeches (186) at the external angle of the eye and at the root of the nose.—Where the swelling is very tenacious: Continual irrigation with permanganate of potassium (1 : 2000).—Wash the everted lids twice a day abundantly with a solution of α-naphtol (0.4 : 1000).

As soon as swelling and false membranes have disappeared: Cauterize with formaldehyde (1 : 500 to 1 : 300) or with nitrate of silver (2 : 100). Repeat daily. [Before using nitrate of silver or formaldehyde solution, clean the whole conjunctival surface very carefully with sublimate (1 : 5000), or, better, with an alumnol solution (4 : 100), which forms with the pus a white precipitate that is very easily removed.]—Linear cauterization of the conjunctival sac with the mitigated pencil (287 *b, d*). Immediately afterwards neutralize with a salt solution. *Do not cauterize again before the scab has fallen off.*— Large granulations should be removed with scissors or cauterized with the unmitigated pencil (287 *b*).

In *unyielding cases:* Replace the nitrate of silver by pure perchloride of hydrogen, or by the iodide of silver *in statu nascendi*, which is obtained by instilling two drops of the following solution:

I. Iodide of potassium	2	30	35 gr.
Distilled water	3	50	53 gr.
Pure glycerin	6	50	100 gr.

and immediately afterwards two drops of the following solution:

II. Crystallized nitrate of silver	3	50	53 gr.
Distilled water	3	50	53 gr.
Pure glycerin	6	50	100 gr.

or try: Daily energetic massage of the whole conjunctiva with calomel.

Should there be any *complication* from the *cornea:* Avoid extra- as well as intra-ocular pressure: Eserine (111) or pilocarpine (251 *a*). [Atropine (23) only in case of central ulcer.]

Besides these therapeutic means, which the physician uses himself, *continual care* should be given to the child *by nurses* remaining with it *day and night.* The nurse will wash the eyes whenever there is the slightest trace of secretion. [Washes with sublimate (1 : 10,000), or salicylate of mercury (1 : 5000), or hydrochinone (2 : 100).]

All *suppuration having ceased*, physician uses boric acid (4 : 100), or a 1 : 200 solution of ammoniated sulphichthyol.—At home an astringent collyrium is used.—Strengthening diet. Act lightly on stools.—Pure air.—High pillow.

70. CONJUNCTIVITIS, CHRONIC.— CHRONIC CATARRH OF THE CONJUNCTIVA.

Keep bowels loose.—Pure fresh air.—Exercise. —Footbaths (118).—Change of climate.—Cold (98 *a*) or Scotch douches (98 *b*).

Avoid: Constipation, liquor, coffee, strong wine, heavy meals, smoke and dust, tiring of eyes, late hours, insomnia (140), but also sleeping too long.

Protection from dust, wind, and strong light by: Coquille lenses, blue or smoked, or veil.

Prohibit caustics and *irritating collyria*. Brush or douche with any of the following solutions: Borate of soda (29), boric acid (30 *a*), yellow astringent collyrium (55), sulphate of zinc (325 *a*), sulphate of copper (80 *a*) [for physician to use], tannic acid (310 *a*), or with:

Salicylic acid	3|0	45 gr.
Biborate of sodium	1|0	15 gr.
Distilled water	500|0	1 pt.

or:

Sulphate of copper . . . } āā 0|02 to 0|04		⅓ gr. to ⅔ gr.
Crystallized alum . . . }		
Distilled water	12|00	℥3
Tincture of opium	0|20	3 gr.
Glycerin	2|00	30 gr.

Eye-douches (99) with thymol (1 : 2000) or benzoate of sodium (3 : 100).

For *itching:* Instillations of cocaine (½ per cent.) and frequent eye-douches with cherry-laurel water.

In case of beginning *excoriations:* oxide of zinc (325 *b*) or white precipitate (229 *d*) ointment.

To *obviate* an *ectropium:* Patient should dry lids, wiping from below upward.

Pull out diseased lashes. Squeeze out Meibomian glands. See that lachrymal ducts are permeable.

Nasal douches (100) or more energetic treatment of coexisting rhinitis (273).

Should the *conjunctivitis resist* all above means of treatment: Repeated abrasions of the epithelial layer of the palpebral conjunctiva with a Desmarres scarificator or any convex scalpel.

71. CONJUNCTIVITIS, CROUPOUS.— PSEUDO-MEMBRANOUS CONJUNCTIVITIS.

Bacteriologic examinations of the false membranes.

For *ordinary cases:* No caustics. Alternating hot and cold compresses moistened with boric acid (3 : 100), carbolic acid (3 : 1000), or permanganate of potassium (1 : 4000). Eye-douches with benzoate of sodium (2 to 4 : 100).

In *tenacious cases:* Remove false membranes and touch up conjunctiva with sublimate (1 : 300) or with nitrate of silver (2 : 100). At the same time vaporize lime water near bed of patient.

In *severe forms* with *fibrinous exudation:* Local treatment of true diphtheritic conjunctivitis (72).

72. CONJUNCTIVITIS, TRUE DIPHTHERITIC.

Vigorous *prophylaxis.* Take all children out of patient's room.—Avoid contact of diphtheritic membranes with mucous membranes.

Antitoxin injection.—Strengthening food. Tonics.—Where necessary, light purgative.—Internally, chloride of iron, 6 drops daily, in milk, or:

Benzoate of sodium	10|0	2½ℨ
Syrup of turpentine	390|0	12½ℨ

Tablespoonful every three hours.

Where one eye alone is attacked: Protect the other [see blennorrhœal conjunctivitis (69)].

Never cauterize in stage of fibrinous infiltration.

Where we find *considerable swelling* and sharp pains: Energetic antiphlogistic treatment [leeches (186) at root of nose and external angle of eye.] *No scarification* of the conjunctiva! [Hardly any blood would flow and the deep tissue would be exposed to the danger of diphtheritic infiltration.]—*Carefully* apply *iced compresses* [circulation being poor there is always danger of necrosis setting in].

As soon as the *swelling subsides:* Replace ice by *hot compresses* to loosen the fibrinous exudation and to hasten absorption. Moisten these compresses with a non-irritating disinfectant: Sublimate 1:10,000, permanganate of potassium 1:4000, benzoate of sodium 2 : 100. Clean eye frequently and carefully.—Vaporize lime water or the following solution near bed of patient :

Rectified oil of turpentine ...... } āā 4|0	āā 1ʒ
Tincture of eucalyptus	
Alcohol .... 300|0	10ʒ
Distilled water .... 1000|0	2 pts

Rub parts covered with false membranes twice daily with a solution of sublimate in glycerin (1 : 100) [wash afterwards with salt water], with lemon-juice, with boric acid (30 *b*), with a solution of chloral 1 : 30 [remove one minute after application with hot water], or with trypsin 10 : 100.

Suppurative stage: Treatment analogous to that of blennorrhœal conjunctivitis (69).—Watch corneal complications (175, 176).

Cicatricial stage: Do not use caustics, and ward off adhesions of the conjunctiva of the lids and the ball of the eye by inserting a probe between the eyeball and the lids daily, and instilling milk, glycerin, or oil into the conjunctival sac.

73. CONJUNCTIVITIS, FOLLICULAR.

Systemic treatment.—Change of climate.—Diet analogous to that of simple conjunctivitis (78). Subacetate of lead (1 to 2 : 100), boric acid (4 : 100), nitrate of silver (1 : 100) [applied only by the physician].—Alum pencil (6 *b*).—Massage with pulverized boric acid (30 *c*).—Smoked glasses.—Nasal douches (100).

74. CONJUNCTIVITIS, GONORRHŒAL, OF ADULTS.

Treatment analogous to that of ophthalmia of the new-born (69), but more vigorous.

75. CONJUNCTIVITIS, GRANULAR.— TRACHOMATOUS CONJUNCTIVITIS.—TRACHOMA.

Rub conjunctiva in its full extent with small pledgets of cotton soaked in the following solution:

Bichloride of mercury	0|50	8 gr.
Chloride of soda	7|00	1 з 45 gr.
Distilled water	1000|00	2 pts.

Repeat rubbing once or twice a day.

Massage of the conjunctiva with boric acid in impalpable powder (30 c) or with powdered calomel (33 c). Afterwards wash with sublimate (1 : 500).—Squeeze out granulations with *roller forceps.*—*Scarifications* parallel with border of lid.—*Cauterizations* with sulphate of copper pencil (80 c) or with alum pencil (6 b).—Brush with a saturated solution of acetate of lead in glycerin.—Cauterize conjunctiva 3 to 4 times a day with chloride of zinc (1 to 2 : 100), not neutralizing afterwards.—Anoint the palpebral conjunctiva with the following glycerole:

Sulphate of copper	0|20	3 gr.
Glycerin ointment	5|00	75 gr.

Where the secretion is great: Cauterize with nitrate of silver (2 : 100).

CONJUNCTIVITIS

In *unyielding cases*, laceration of the mucous membrane with a metallic brush.—Remove excrescences. Excision of the fold of transmission.—Cauterize repeatedly with the galvano-cautery. [In the intervals: Massage with iodol vaseline 10 : 100.]—Electrolysis [30 m. a. until quite a little foam has formed; previous to this, incisions into the palpebral conjunctiva].

In *desperate cases:* Transplantation of conjunctiva or of mucous membrane of the oral cavity.

Abundant washes at home with sublimate 1: 5000 or sulphate of copper (80 *a*).

Vary the treatments, combine them, adapt to each special case.

Have these *two important rules* in your mind always:

I. Turn the upper lid well, using, when necessary, torsion forceps, and treat the upper conjunctival sac in its whole extent, the corners included, the internal and external angles being the principal seat of the granulations.

II. Never cause a loss of conjunctival or subconjunctival tissue. Limit yourself to achieve a modification of tissue.

Treatment of *trachomatous pannus:* Direct massage of the cornea with boric acid finely pulverized (30 *c*) or with aristol.—Peritomy or careful galvano-cauterization of the limbus.—Repeated abrasion of the epithelial layer of palpebral conjunctiva with a Desmarres scarificator or a lance with blunt point.—Where pannus does not yield: Try *careful* application of a maceration of *old* jequirity seeds (165) three times a day until considerable secretion and swelling have been produced.

Treatment of *complications:* Ulcers of the cornea (176) [do not scrape], complications from lachrymal apparatus (91, 180, 181), ectropion (103), or entropion (106), distichiasis (97), symblepharon (306).

Systemic treatment: Change of air, country life.—Good nourishment.—Avoid congestions.—Tonics [iron (164), iodine (147 *b*), arsenic (20)].—Medicinal baths (25 *c, d, e*).

Conjunctivitis, Phlyctenular. *See* PHLYCTENULAR KERATITIS (173).

76. CONJUNCTIVITIS PRODUCED BY ATROPINE.

Examine collyrium as to its being sterilized.—Where necessary replace atropine by duboisine (102) or scopolamin (284).—Eye-douche with non-irritating collyria [see simple conjunctivitis (78)].

77. CONJUNCTIVITIS, PURULENT (not blennorrhœal).

Sublimate (1 : 500), formalin (119), or pure peroxide of hydrogen (135). Applications to be made *by the physician.*

At home: Sublimate (1 : 5000).

Where swelling is great: Iced compresses.

As soon as suppuration has ceased: Treat as simple conjunctivitis (78).

78. CONJUNCTIVITIS, SIMPLE, Catarrhal.—CATARRH OF CONJUNCTIVA.

Keep bowels loose.—*Avoid* bad air, smoke (above all, tobacco smoke), radiating heat, congestions to the head, all work tiring the eyes.

Smoked glasses.—Examine conjunctiva for foreign bodies; remove them.

Brush conjunctiva, douche the eye and wash with one of the following collyria: Boric acid (30 *a*), biborate of sodium (29), yellow astringent collyrium (55), sulphate of zinc (325 *a*), subacetate of lead (185 *a*).

For *pain:* Add to the collyrium some drops of tincture of opium or try a combination of boric acid and cocaine, as follows:

Boric acid	5|0	75 gr.
Muriate of cocaine	1|0	15 gr.
Distilled water	125|0	4 $\bar{3}$
Cherry-laurel water	25|0	6½ $\bar{3}$

Should there be considerable *swelling* of the lids: Compresses with subacetate of lead solution (185 *d*) or iced water.

In *unyielding cases:* Brush the palpebral conjunctiva every other day with a solution of nitrate of silver (0|5 to 1:100), provided there is much secretion. Where, however, there is no or hardly any secretion but swelling of the follicles: Careful cauterization with the blue pencil (80 *c'''*) [in sensitive patients pulverized calomel stops pain promptly].

As a general rule, *repeated use of a weak remedy is to be preferred to the application of a strong one.*

Watch the border of the lids. *See* BLEPHARITIS (26).

Where necessary: Reopen lachrymal passages by simple probing.

79. CONJUNCTIVITIS, VERNAL.—VERNAL CATARRH.

As a rule: No irritants, no astringents. Washes and compresses of carbolized water (1:500), or salicylic acid (1:200), or boric acid (2:100).—Massage with calomel ointment (33 *a*) or cocaine ointment (52 *b*).

Exceptionally, where there is no improvement by above treatment: Instillations of acetic acid (1:100) four times a day. Where there is considerable proliferation of conjunctival tissue: Excision of the hypertrophied parts on the level of the conjunctiva and the corneal limbus. Galvano-cautery.

Glasses to protect the eyes.—Hygienic diet.—*Change of climate.*

80. COPPER, SULPHATE OF.

a. Sulphate of copper . . . . 0|60   8 gr.
    Rose water   . . . . 50|00   1ʒ 53
    Distilled water. . . . . 150|00   5ʒ
       Dissolve and filter.

b. Sulphate of copper . . . . 1|0   15 gr.
    Glycerin . . . . 10|0   2½ʒ

c. Crystallized sulphate of copper.
c′. Pure crystal — unmitigated blue stick.
c″. Sulphate of copper . . . . } Equal parts = mitigated
    Nitrate of potassium . . . }   blue stick.

c'''. Crystallized sulphate of copper ⎫
Nitrate of potassium . . . . ⎬ Equal parts = divine stone.
Alum . . . . ⎭

81. CORNEA, ABSCESS OF THE.

Treat as infected ulcer (176).—Prevent spontaneous perforation by puncture with cautery.

Cornea, Burns of the. *See* BURNS OF THE CONJUNCTIVA (57).

82. CORNEA, CALCAREOUS CONCRETIONS OF THE.

Remove with sharp spoon or small gouge. Antiseptic bandage.

83. CORNEA, FISTULA OF THE.

Freshen up edges. Eserine (111) or atropine (23 *a*), according to seat of fistula (peripheral or central). Antiseptic pressure bandage (101).

84. CORNEA, FOREIGN BODY OF THE.

On anterior *surface* of cornea: *Try in all cases to remove with brush.* Where unsuccessful with brush try Daviel's spoon. Exceptionally: Cauterize carefully with galvano-cautery, and try several days later to remove the foreign body with the scab.

Where foreign body penetrates deeply into the *corneal tissue:* Introduce cataract-needle behind it and remove.

Where foreign body has penetrated into *anterior chamber:* Paracentesis and extraction with iridectomy forceps or with the magnet.

Where foreign body has penetrated into the *tissue* of the *iris:* Iridectomy.

85. CORNEA, HERPES OF THE.—HERPETIC KERATITIS.

Dry aseptic bandage. Boric acid ointment (30 *d*).

In unyielding cases: Destroy the vesicles by massage, with a sufficient quantity of powdered calomel. Thereupon treatment analogous to that of ulcerous keratitis (176).

For pain: Instillations of cocaine (52 *a*) and injections of morphine (231 *c*) into the preauricular region.

86. CORNEA, LESIONS OF THE.

Remove foreign body. In perforating wounds: Eserine (111) where perforation is peripheral; atropine (23 *a*) where it is central.

Iris having prolapsed: Ablation with scissors or destruction with galvano-cautery of the herniated part. *Strict antisepsis,* sublimate (1 : 5000) dressing.

87. CORNEA, LEUCOMA OF THE.—FILM OF THE CORNEA.—NEPHELION.

According to time of subsistence and age of individual: Calomel ointment (33 *a*), red precipitate ointment (229 *c*), yellow oxide ointment (229 *b*), or blue ointment:

Blue ointment	1|0	15 gr.
Yellow vaseline	2|0	30 gr.
Lanolin	1|0	15 gr.

[*Blue ointment alone is too great an irritant.*]

Direct steaming of the anæsthetized cornea. Insufflation of calomel (33 c) or boric acid (30 c), followed by massage.

Try: *Electrolysis*, 3 to 4 m. a., until foam forms upon the surface of the cornea. Duration of application, ½ to 2 minutes once a week. Or direct galvanization for several weeks daily 1 to 3 minutes; ½ to 1½ m. a., just as patient tolerates it.

Or yet (but *only* in *fresh cases*): *Subconjunctival injections* of tepid *salt water* [salt, 1|0 to 3|0 (15 gr. to 45 gr.); sterilized water, 30|0 (1ℨ)] near the corneal border; whereupon massage and pressure bandage. Or use:

Sulphate of cadmium	0|05	⅚ gr.
Distilled water	4|00	1ℨ
Gum arabic	2|00	30 gr.
Extract of opium	0|10	1½ gr.

Apply with a brush to centre of the leucoma.

Where vision is bettered by mydriasis: *Iridectomy.* The place of this iridectomy and its size will vary with the situation and extent of the leucoma.

Tattooing with india-ink in antiseptic solution.

Abrasion where there are calcareous incrustations or deposits of metallic salts (acetate of lead, nitrate of silver).

For fresh corneal opacities produced by slaked lime: Instillation of a sugar solution, which changes the lime into a soluble saccharate.

Vision in irregular astigmatism is bettered with stenopæic glasses. *See*, furthermore, Nos. 22 *b* and 177.

88. CORNEA, ADHERENT LEUCOMA OF THE.

Iridectomy, to better vision and to combat inflammation. Careful tattooing.

89. CORNEA, TUMORS OF THE.

Remove them. Antiseptic bandage.
Larger malignant tumors: Enucleation.

Cornea, Ulcer of the. *See* ULCEROUS KERATITIS (176).

90. CYCLITIS.—IRIDOCYCLITIS.

Rest, atropine (23 *a*), poultices (255), diaphoresis (305), purgatives, smoked glasses.—For the pain: Morphine (231 *c*), strengthening treatment, iron (164) and iodine (147) preparations.—In case of synechiæ: Iridectomy as soon as inflammation has subsided.

Cysticercus. *See* CYSTICERCUS OF CONJUNCTIVA (58) and C. OF VITREOUS (319).

Dacryocystitis, Acute. *See* PURULENT DACRYOCYSTITIS (92).

91. DACRYOCYSTITIS, CHRONIC.

Squeeze out contents of lachrymal sac, make an injection and see whether the liquid escapes through the nose. If not, dilate lachrymal canaliculi with a conical probe, and introduce into the nasal canal an olive button probe.—Where there is a stricture: Split *one* of the canaliculi (the *upper* one *in preference*).

DACRYOCYSTITIS

Methodical probing.—Where there is total obstruction of the nasal canal open a passage by force with Weber's knife.

Each probing is to be followed by an injection of boric acid (4 : 100), or sublimate (1 : 3000), or permanganate of potassium (1 : 1000), or with one of the following solutions:

Boric acid	10|00	2½ʒ
Salicylic acid	2|50	38 gr.
Distilled water	500|00	1 pt.

Triturated iodoform	10|0 to 25|0	2½ʒ to 6½ʒ
Glycerin . . . . . . } āā	40|0	āā 1ʒ 2½ʒ
Distilled water . . . . }		

Shake solution before each injection.

In *unyielding* cases give probes a coating of

Triturated iodoform or iodol	5|0	75 gr.
Cocoa butter	30|0	1ʒ

Where dacryocystitis resists all these forms of treatment, or where patient has but a few days to spare for treatment: Perform a *curettage* of the lachrymal sac and naso-lachrymal canal with a small curved sharp fenestrated spoon.

Where the lachrymal sac is much dilated: Partial resection of the anterior wall of the sac.

Where coexisting *fistula of the lachrymal sac* does not disappear with the re-establishment of the lachrymal passages: Use of *galvano-cautery* or *excision* of the *membrane* lining the fistulous duct and careful suture of the margins of the wound.

Coexisting conjunctivitis (70, 75, 78), rhinitis (273), syphilis (291), or tuberculosis requires special treatment.

92. DACRYOCYSTITIS, PURULENT.—PHLEGMON OF THE LACHRYMAL SAC.

Slit *both* canaliculi up to the lachrymal sac. Cut through the internal ligament with scissors to unite both wounds, and thus open the superior part of the sac completely.—Squeeze out contents.—Instil several drops of tincture of iodine or cauterize with mitigated pencil (287 *b, d*) [prevent injected liquid getting into eye].

Inject lachrymal sac with sublimate (3 : 1000), chloride of zinc ($\frac{1}{2}$ to 1 : 100), creolin (2 to 4 : 100), thymol (0.05 to 1 : 1000) (312), sulphocarbolate of zinc (1 to 3 : 100), or phenosalyl (4 : 1000).

Where inflammation is very great: Permanganate of potassium (2 : 1000).

Injections should be *very carefully* made, on account of *danger* from *periorbital phlegmon*.

In the interval patient should empty lachrymal sac frequently by squeezing. Sublimate compresses (1 : 5000), or boric acid (4 : 100), or subacetate of lead solution (185 *d*).

Acute symptoms having disappeared: Probe nasal canal and treat as in chronic dacryocystitis (91).

93. DACRYOPS.

Excision of a part of the wall of the cyst and closure of the wound by sutures.

94. DALTONISM.—PARTIAL ACHROMATOPSIS.

In slight degrees of partial achromatopsis: Try glasses colored with fuchsin that increases the difference between red and green.

A color-blind person should never take up a calling which necessitates his being perfectly able to distinguish between colors, as: Coast-guard, sailor, switchman, dyer, dealer in or manufacturer of colored cloth.

95. DERMATOL.—BASIC GALLATE OF BISMUTH.

Can sometimes take the place of iodoform. Has no odor and does not irritate.

Dermatol		1|0	15 gr.
Oxide of zinc . . . . } āā	6|0	1½З
Starch			
Vaseline		12|0	3З

Mix and make a paste.

For eczema of the lids.

Diastase. *See* EXTRACT OF MALT (115).

96. DIGITALIS.

Powdered digitalis leaves	0|10	1½ gr.
White sugar	0|40	6½ gr.

3 to 5 powders a day.

97. DISTICHIASIS.

Transplantation of ciliary margin.

Electrolysis: A fine platin-iridium needle, made

expressly for this purpose, is attached to the negative pole, while the positive electrode rests upon the arm. Strength of current can be increased to 8 m. a. Duration: A few seconds. *Decrease slowly to zero.* The lashes may be pulled out or left to fall out by themselves.—Remove but a few lashes at one time, and *protect* the *cocainized eye* by a plate of horn.

98. DOUCHES.

a. Cold douche: 8° to 10° C. [47° to 50° F.]; short. Begin with douche of 3 seconds, and do not apply longer than 25 or 30 seconds.

b. Scottish douche: Begin with hot douche of 30° C. [86° F.], increase temperature to 35°, 40°, and 45° C. [95°, 104°, and 113° F.], and end with a cold stream of 8° C. [47° F.].

c. Alternating douche: Alternating hot and cold stream, for an equal number of seconds (10 to 15); not longer than 2 minutes altogether.

All douches can be thrown as a *spray* or a *stream*. On the whole, the stream is to be preferred. Direct it principally along the vertebral column, on feet, calves, and legs.

Whichever form of douche is used patient should observe the *following rules:*

Take a short walk before the douche.

Protect head and contract muscles during douche.

Dress quickly, and take vigorous exercise after douche (horseback-riding, gymnastics, fencing, etc.).

99. DOUCHES, EYE-DOUCHES.

a. Steam-douche to clear up fresh corneal opacities. The cornea is steamed directly, and where necessary, protected by a thin muslin bandage. Time: 15 to 30 minutes.

b. Simple spray: Patient opens and closes eye, exposing conjunctiva as much as possible. Dry the eye carefully after spray. Any appropriate collyrium can be used as a spray. Time: 30 to 40 seconds.

c. As a quite *strong stream* in cases of asthenopia of neurasthenic origin. Apply to ocular and frontal region, the eyes remaining closed; dry, and use massage afterwards.

100. DOUCHE, NASAL.

Place vessel containing liquid about 50 centimetres (½ yard) above the head.—Insert olive of canula horizontally, so that one nostril is completely closed by it.—Hold the *head erect*, having care to *breathe* with *open mouth* to hinder liquid from penetrating into pharynx, and let it run out of the other nostril.—Douche through one nostril after the other.—After douche *wait* at least *20 minutes before blowing nose.*

101. DRESSING, ANTISEPTIC.

Solutions for eye-baths:

Corrosive sublimate	0|20	3 gr.
Distilled water	1000|00	2 pts.

Patient washes, brushes, and disinfects his hands, soaks small pieces of hygroscopic cotton in the solution and places them upon the eye, which has been previously covered with a bit of muslin cut round, moistened with sublimate.—A strip of oiled silk, or gutta-percha tissue-paper, overlapping the cotton on all sides, hinders evaporation.—Dressing is held in place by a muslin or fine linen bandage.

Where patient cannot tolerate the sublimate, replace it by boric acid (30 *a* or 30 *b*).

Drooping of the Upper Lid. *See* PTOSIS (258).

102. DUBOISINE.

Neutral sulphate of duboisine	00|05	$\frac{3}{8}$ gr.
Distilled water	10|00	$2\frac{1}{3}$

Instil one drop several times a day.

Duboisine combined with atropine. *See* ATROPINE (23 *c*).

Ecchymosis. *See* CONJUNCTIVA (59) and LIDS (196).

103. ECTROPION.

Cauterize with galvano-cautery.—Surgical treatment.

Eczema of the Cornea. *See* PHLYCTENULAR KERATITIS (173).

Effusion of Blood into Anterior Chamber. *See* HYPHÆMA (138).

104. EMBOLISM OF CENTRAL ARTERY.

Careful massage of the eyeball. Repeated paracentesis of the anterior chamber.—Atropine (23 *a*). Keep bowels loose.—Avoid every excess (on account of the other eye).

105. EMPHYSEMA, SUBCONJUNCTIVAL.

Etiological treatment.—Pressure bandage.

106. ENTROPION.

Cauterize with galvano-cautery.—Surgical treatment.

107. EPICANTHUS.

Surgical treatment not before the eighth or the tenth year. The development of the nasal bone makes this anomaly either disappear or modifies it in all cases.

108. EPISCLERITIS.

Protect the eye: Dark glasses, or, better, a *dry* bandage.—Apply *dry* heat: Aromatic leaves (255 *f*) or conium leaves (255 *g*) in linen bags heated and applied to the eye for hours.—Massage with cocaine ointment (52 *b*), calomel ointment or powder (33 *a, c*).

For acute pain and pericorneal injection: Instil combined atropine and cocaine collyrium (23 *b*).

For coexisting conjunctivitis: Hot eye-baths with boric acid (30 *a*) or borate of sodium (29). Afterwards dry the eye thoroughly.

Watch the general health.

109. ERGOTIN.

As the different preparations of ergotin are of very variable strength, it is *better to prescribe ergotinin*, the alkaloid itself.

Ergotinin . . . . 0|02   ⅓ gr.
Sugar of milk . . . . 0|50   8 gr.
Liquorice powder q. s.
 To make 50 pills; 3 pills daily.

110. EROSIONS (OR FISSURES) AT THE OUTER ANGLE OF THE EYE.

Ichthyol . . . . 4|0   15
Lanolin . . . .⎫ āā 5|0   75 gr.
Glycerin . . . .⎭
Olive oil . . . . 1|0   15 gr.

Repeated application with the pure or mitigated pencil of nitrate of silver (287 *b*).

111. ESERINE OR PHYSOSTIGMINE.

Neutral sulphate of eserine . . 0|03 to 00|10   ½ gr. to 1½ gr.
Distilled water   . . . .   10|00   2½3
 Instil one drop several times a day.

112. ETHER.

a. Pure ether. Sulphuric ether.
 Hypodermic injections in case of collapse produced by chloroform.
 Pravaz syringeful several times.

b. Hypodermic injection of *camphorated ether:*
 Camphor . . . . 1 part,
 Ether . . . . 4 to 5 parts,
has a stronger effect than sulphuric ether alone.

Ether as a *narcotic. See* CHLOROFORM ANÆSTHESIA (42).

113. ETHYL BROMIDE.

Anæsthetic for a *short narcosis.*—Inhalation of 10|0 to 15|0 (2½5 to 45); maximal dose 20|0 (55).

It is dangerous to narcotize an individual twice on same day with this anæsthetic.

Pure ethyl bromide is colorless, completely transparent; odor and taste is similar to ether.

114. EXALGIN (METHYLACETANILID).

Exalgin	2|50	38 gr.
Spirits of peppermint	10|00	2½ʒ
Aqua tiliæ	120|00	4ʒ
Syrup of orange flowers	15|00	4ʒ

Tablespoonful several times a day.

Exophthalmic Goitre. *See* GOITRE (129*A*).

115. EXTRACT OF MALT.

2 teaspoonfuls twice a day.—Give preference to *diastase*, a powder of which 0|5 to 1|0 (7 gr. to 15 gr.) should be taken three times a day.

Eyelashes, Loss of the. *See* LOSS OF THE EYELASHES (226).

116. FIORAVENTI, BALSAM OF.

Cinnamon oil; clove oil; juniper oil; mace oil; turpentine oil; thyme oil	gtt. 5
Peru balsam	gtt. 4
Alcohol . . . . 100|0	3ʒ 2ʒ

Rub on forehead and temples.

Fissures. *See* EROSIONS (110).

Fistula of the Lachrymal Sac. *See* under the heading of CHRONIC DACRYOCYSTITIS (91).

117. FLUORESCIN.

Fluorescin	00|40	6½ gr.
Carbonate of sodium	00|70	11 gr.
Distilled water	20|00	5ℨ

Instil 1 drop, close the eye for several seconds, and wash with any collyrium.

Stains the parts of the cornea bare of epithelium green and those of the conjunctiva yellow.—Where epithelium is only altered the stain will be less marked.

118. FOOT-BATHS, MEDICATED.

Take foot-baths of an evening before supper or 2 or 3 hours after supper. 5 to 7 quarts of water. —Time, 20 seconds to 2 minutes.—Wipe feet, and dry them thoroughly by rubbing afterwards. Temperature, 35° to 40° C. [95° to 104° F.].

a. Mustard foot-bath. Foot-bath with mustard flour :

Mix 125|0 (4ℨ) of mustard flour with cold or barely lukewarm water. Add later a sufficient quantity of water.—Be careful not to put in any vinegar.

b. Hydrochlorate of Ammonium foot-bath :

Hydrochlorate of ammonium	250|0	8ℨ
Water q. s. for a foot-bath.		

c. Acid foot-bath :

Muriatic acid	120|0 to 150|0	4ℨ to 5ℨ
Water q. s. for a foot-bath.		

d. Alkaline foot-bath :

Carbonate of sodium	125|0	4ℨ
Water q. s. for a foot-bath.		

c. Sea-Salt foot-bath :

Sea-salt	125|0	4ʒ
Water q. s. for a foot-bath.		

Formaldehyde. *See* FORMALIN (119).

119. FORMALIN.–FORMIC ALDEHYDE. –FORMOL.

a. For disinfecting instruments: solution 1 : 500.
b. For the conjunctiva: solution 1 : 2000.
c. In blenorrhœa increase strength of solution up to 1 : 300.

Fowler's Solution. *See* ARSENIC (20 *a*).

120. GALLANOL.—GALLIC ACID ANILIDE.

Gallanol	1|0 to 4|0	15 gr. to	1ʒ
Vaseline	20|0	5	ʒ

Cover with **traumaticin** (*10 per cent. solution of gutta-percha in chloroform*).

Eczema of the eyelids.

121. GELSEMIUM.

Tincture of gelsemium sempervirens.
15 to 30 drops several times a day on a piece of sugar.

Neuralgia of the fifth nerve and spasm of the orbicular muscle.

122. GLAND, LACHRYMAL, FISTULA OF THE.

Freshen up edges and close fistula by sutures. Cauterization.

123. GLAND, LACHRYMAL, INFLAMMATION OF THE.

Poultices (255).—Where there is fluctuation: Incision through conjunctiva.

124. GLAND, LACHRYMAL, TUMORS OF THE.

Extirpation.

125. GLASSES FOR WORK, RULES FOR PRESCRIBING.

1. Establish necessary refraction for distinct vision at working distance (t). It is in inverse ratio to this distance.

Example: For 25 cm., or $\frac{100 \text{ cm.}}{4}$: $t = 4$ D.

2. Establish the amplitude of accommodation or dynamic refraction (a), of which *only two-thirds* $\left(\frac{2a}{3}\right)$ should be used for work, while one-third remains as a reserve. (*The following table* shows the normal amplitude of accommodation for different ages.)

Example: For the age of 40: $a = 4.5$ D; therefore $\frac{2a}{3} = 3$ D.

3. Establish the maximum of refraction which can be used for work (u) by adding the two-thirds of the dynamic refraction to the static refraction (r); $u = \frac{2a}{3} + r$. In myopia r is plus; in hypermetropia it is minus.

GLASSES

4. *The glass for work (w) is found by subtracting the maximum of usable refraction for working distance (u) from the necessary refraction (t)*: $W = t - u$.

In our example (age 40, working distance 25 cm.):

$W = 4 - 3 = 1$ for the emmetropic eye (where $r = o$).

$W = 4 - (3 - 2.5) = 3.5$ for the hypermetropic eye of 2.5 D. (r negative).

$W = 4 - (3 + 0.75) = 0.25$ for the myopic eye of 0.75 D. (r positive).

We should remark that the myopic eye but rarely needs the help of concave glasses for work this side of its far point.

YEARS.	Amplitude of accommodation according to Donders. a.	$\frac{a}{3}$	Usable accommodation in round numbers. $\frac{2a}{3}$
10	14	4.7	9
15	12	4	8
20	10	3.3	6.5
25	8.5	2.8	5.5
30	7	2.3	4.5
35	5.5	1.83	3.5
40	4.5	1.5	3
45	3.5	1.17	2.5
50	2.5	0.83	1.75
55	1.75	0.58	1.25
60	1	0.33	0.75
65	0.75	0.25	0.5
70	0.25	0.08	0

See also PRESBYOPIA (256).

126. GLAUCOMA, ABSOLUTE.

Where there are violent attacks with irritation of the other eye : Enucleation.

127. GLAUCOMA, ACUTE.

Forbid mydriatics and poultices.

Eserine (111). *pilocarpine* (251 *a*). Drastic cathartics, diuresis, and diaphoresis (305). Complete rest of body and mind. Bloodletting (186). Narcotics, hypodermic injections of morphine (231 *c*).

Repeated *paracentesis*. *Iridectomy* from above. Large and peripheral incision. [Where the tension is great iridectomy can be facilitated by making a puncture of the sclera first.] *Anterior sclerotomy:* Puncture and counter-puncture as much in the periphery as possible [should about correspond with the horizontal meridian] ; push the knife up as high as possible on both sides, but leave a bridge of sclera separating cuts to prevent prolapse of the iris. Sclerotomy with the lance, repeated at diverse points of the limbus. *Posterior sclerotomy:* Incision at region of the equator of the eye between rectus externus and rectus superior ; let a little of the vitreous escape.

Always regulate the outflow of aqueous humor or vitreous carefully in order to prevent intra-ocular hemorrhages.

After the operation : Instil myotics (235) repeatedly.

128. GLAUCOMA, CHRONIC.

Myotics (235).—Avoid congestions to the head and excitement.—Iridectomy.—Incision of the angle of the iris.—Anterior or posterior sclerotomy. For pain: Narcotics.

129. GLAUCOMA, HEMORRHAGIC.

Rest.—Myotics (235).—Ice.—For pain: Narcotics, exceptionally lukewarm poultices with conium leaves (255 *g*), hypodermic injections of morphine (231 *c*).—*Punctures* through the sclera, *do not try any other operations.*—Where pain persists: Enucleation.

129*A*. GOITRE, EXOPHTHALMIC.— GRAVES' DISEASE.—BASEDOW'S DISEASE.

Phosphate of sodium in doses of 15|0 (½ȝ) *pro die.* Preparations of *thyroidin* (daily dose should represent 2|0 to 4|0 [⅓ȝ to 1ȝ] of the fresh gland.) Cease giving thyroidin as soon as diarrhœa sets in or where there is no amelioration of symptoms after three weeks of this treatment. Galvanization of the cervical sympathetic nerve. Hydrotherapy (98). Light diet. Avoid mental emotions as much as possible. In severe and unyielding cases extirpation of the cervical sympathetic.

Granulations. *See* GRANULAR CONJUNCTIVITIS (75).

Graves' Disease. *See* EXOPHTHALMIC GOITRE (129*A*).

130. HEBRA'S OINTMENT.

Simple lead plaster . . . . } āā 10|0	2½ȝ
Olive oil	

Spread on piece of linen; renew application every 24 hours at least.

131. HEMERALOPIA RESULTING FROM TORPOR OF THE RETINA.

Systemic treatment.—Treat gastric and intestinal troubles. Strengthening food, open air, gymnastic exercises.—Quinine (259), iron (164), cod-liver oil (54).—Keep patient away from noxious influences [excess of work, strong light].—Prescribe smoked glasses and instil myotics (235) in a weak solution for a long time.—Correct with glasses anomalies of refraction.

132. HEMIANOPSIA.—HEMIOPIA.

Etiologic treatment.—In case of apoplexy: Derivative treatment; absolute rest; elevated position of head; ice bag; later electricity.

133. HOMATROPINE.

Hydrobromate or sulphate of
homatropine . . . . 0|1 to 0|3   1½ gr. to 4½ gr.
Distilled water . . . .   10|0   2$\frac{1}{15}$

Instil from 2 to 4 drops, at 5 minutes' interval between drops. To determine refraction.

Hordeolum. *See* STYE (301).

134. HYDRASTIS CANADENSIS.

Fluid extract of hydrastis canadensis.
Several times daily 10 to 15 drops.

Hydrochloric Acid. *See* FOOT-BATHS (118 c).

135. HYDROGEN, PEROXIDE OF.—OXYGENATED WATER.

a. Pure peroxide of hydrogen, 3 per cent., which means having 3 per cent. of its weight of oxygen.

For antiseptic dressings, principally in purulent processes of conjunctiva and cornea.

b. Pure peroxide of hydrogen, 2 to 3 per cent. . 40|0 1ʒ 2½ʓ
Vaseline . . . . 20|0 5ʓ
Lanolin . . . . 10|0 2½ʓ
(Unna's ointment.)

Hydrophthalmos. *See* CHRONIC GLAUCOMA (128).

Hydrotherapy. *See* DOUCHES (98).

136. HYOSCINE.

Hydrochlorate of hyoscine . . . . 00|01 ⅙ gr.
Distilled water . . . . 20|00 2½ʓ

One syringeful $= 0|0005$ ($\frac{1}{125}$ gr.) *of hyoscine; do not inject more than* $0|001$ ($\frac{1}{60}$ gr.). *See* also MYDRIATICS (233).

Hyoscyamine. *See* HYOSCINE (136).

Hyoscyamus, Oil of. *See* BALSAMUM TRANQUILLANS (24).

137. HYPERMETROPIA.

Judicious use of convex lenses should the asthenopia or insufficiency of vision demand it. For *distant vision*, correct at most but the manifest hypermetropia.

In choosing a glass for *near vision* it is well to remember that *only* ⅔ of the amplitude of accommodation are to be used for continuous work, so that a reserve of ⅓ remains. Therefore *a lens relieving ⅓ of the amplitude of accommodation should be prescribed.*

Example: Hyp. $= 0.75$. Ampl. of acc. $= 3$.
Working distance, ⅓ metre.

We have, therefore, a postulate for a positive power of refraction of $0.75 + 4 = 4.75$ D. Patient supplies ⅔ of his amplitude of accommodation $= 2$ D. He lacks $4.75 - 2 = 2.75$ D. which has to be prescribed in the form of the convex glass.

Therefore + 2.75 D is the reading glass in our example.

For ordinary reading distance, *see* table of PRESBYOPIA (256).

When there is a *tendency to convergent strabismus* prescribe *stronger glasses*. *See* CONVERGENT STRABISMUS (295).

The troublesome *prismatic effect* of strong convex lenses can be neutralized by decentring them, or by a combination of the convex glass with a prism basis inward. For near and far vision without a change of spectacles: *Franklin glasses* or *bifocals*.

In *aphakia:* Prescribe for distance a glass correcting entire hypermetropia; for near vision add to this the lens corresponding to the distance wanted.

Example: Hyp. 11 corrected by + 11.0 D. For vision at ⅓ m. add + 3, thus making it 14 D in all.

138. HYPHÆMA.

Etiologic treatment.—Aid resorption by compresses with subacetate of lead solution (185 *d*), and pressure bandage or massage with cocaine ointment (52 *b*).—Where there are symptoms of *irritation* [pericorneal injection, severe pains] due to a larger effusion of blood: *Paracentesis* made at the lower margin of the cornea. Let the blood escape very slowly, compressing the globe gently through the upper lid to ward off the danger of renewed hemorrhages *ex vacuo*.

139. ICHTHYOL.

Ichthyol	3|0	45 gr.
White vaseline	20|0	5ʒ

140. INSOMNIA.

Sleep with head lowered. Well-aired bedroom. Lukewarm bath and warm milk before retiring. Pillow stuffed with hops.—Bromides (31), chloral hydrate (39), sulphonal (303), trional (315), lactophenin (183).

141. INSTILLING OF COLLYRIA.

Instil with an eye-dropper.—Avoid touching conjunctiva with eye-dropper.—After instillation keep eye closed from 3 to 5 minutes.—Compress lachrymal passages where there is danger from a poisonous collyrium.

142. INSUFFICIENCY OF CONVERGENCE.

Refrain from work which tires the eye.—Aid vision (correct astigmatism).—Strengthen the general system.

Methodical and moderate *exercise* of *convergence*: Simple, well-defined object (black line on white background, luminous slit of Landolt's dynamometer). Patient brings object slowly nearer in median axis as long as he can keep simple binocular vision.

Where insufficiency is of *slight degree* [1 or 2 metre angles (see table hereafter)]: Prescribe *prisms*, base inward, which can be combined with glasses permitting near work.

Should this treatment prove to be *ineffectual*: *Advancement* of *one* of the *internal* recti muscles. If after weeks and months the *insufficiency* still *per*-

INSUFFICIENCY OF CONVERGENCE

sists: *Advancement* of the *internal* rectus of the *other eye*. *Tenotomy of an external rectus is permissible only where power of divergence is very great* (more than 1 metre angle), as it nearly always loses more for the eye in excursion on the side of the operated muscle than it gains on the opposite side.—By advancement we gain much more for the operated side without causing any loss on the other.—Therefore with a *tenotomy* we can bring about a vexatious *insufficiency* of *divergence* (conv. strabismus with homonymous diplopia) *without correcting* the *insufficiency* of *convergence*, which is not to be feared in an advancement.

TABLE SHOWING REDUCTION

OF DEGREES INTO METRE ANGLES [M. A.]		OF METRE ANGLES [M. A.] INTO DEGREES.	
Basis Line.* 58 mm.	Basis Line.* 64 mm.	Basis Line.* 58 mm.	Basis Line.* 64 mm.
Degrees. M. A.	Degrees. M. A.	M. A. Degrees.	M. A. Degrees.
0.5° = 0.3	0.5° = 0.27	0.5 = 0.50°	0.5 = 0.55°
1° = 0.6	1° = 0.55	1 = 1.40°	1 = 1.50°
1.50° = 0.9	1.50° = 0.82	2 = 3.20°	2 = 3.40°
2° = 1.2	2° = 1.09	3 = 5°	3 = 5.30°
2.50° = 1.5	2.50° = 1.36	4 = 6.40°	4 = 7.20°
3° = 1.8	3° = 1.64	5 = 8.20°	5 = 9.10°
4° = 2.4	4° = 2.18	6 = 10°	6 = 11°
5° = 3.0	5° = 2.73	7 = 11.40°	7 = 12.50°
6° = 3.6	6° = 3.27	8 = 13.20°	8 = 14.40°
7° = 4.2	7° = 3.82	9 = 15°	9 = 16.30°
8° = 4.8	8° = 4.36	10 = 16.40°	10 = 18.20°
9° = 5.4	9° = 4.91	11 = 18.20°	11 = 20.10°
10° = 6.0	10° = 5.45	12 = 20°	12 = 22°

* *As basis line the distance between the centres of rotation of the two eyes is designated.*

143. INUNCTIONS, MERCURIAL. — INUNCTIONS WITH BLUE OINTMENT.

Simple mercurial ointment [*1 part mercury to 2 parts excipient*].

Prescribe 10 packages of 2|0 (½ℨ) wrapped in oiled paper.—Rub contents of one package into a different part of the body each day: Left calf, right calf, left thigh, right thigh, left forearm, right forearm. Rub well into skin (15 minutes). Take a lukewarm bath every four days. Rinse the mouth frequently, and brush teeth with:

Chlorate of potassium	10|0	2½ℨ
Distilled water	500|0	1 pt.

For *more energetic* mercurial treatment, *see* SPECIFIC TREATMENT (291).

144. INUNCTIONS, SOOTHING.

a.
Conicine	0|01 to 00|03	⅙ gr. to ½ gr.
Alcohol	50|00	1ℨ 5ℨ

b.
Balsamum tranquillans	20|00	5ℨ
Chloroform	10|00	2½ℨ
Tincture of opium	5|00	75 gr.
Fluid extract belladonna	} āā 0|50	āā 7½ gr.
Fluid extract hyoscyamus		

Shake before using.

145. INUNCTIONS, STIMULATING.

a. With bay rum
b. Spirits of camphor.
c. Balsam of Fioraventi (116).
    Spirits of peppermint } āā 50|0 āā 1ℨ 5ℨ
    Spirits of rosemary

146. IODIDE OF POTASSIUM.

Ointments:

a. Iodide of potassium . . . . 2|0   ½ʒ
   Benzoinated lard . . . . 20|0   5ʒ

b. Iodide of potassium . . . . 2|00   ½ʒ
   Pure iodine . . . . 0|50   8 gr.
   Benzoinated lard . . . . 20|00   5ʒ

   Inunctions of forehead and temples once to twice daily.

c. *Syrup* iodide of potassium:

Iodide of potassium . . . . 10|0   2½ʒ
Syrup of orange peel . . . . 50|0   1ℨ 5ʒ
Distilled water . . . . 250|0   8ℨ

One tablespoonful at least one-half hour before meals.

147. IODINE.

a. *Tincture* of iodine (use preferably the tincture from which color has been removed by ammonia; it has the same action).

External use: Frictions and applications.
Internal use: 15 to 20 drops in half a glass of iced milk in obstinate vomiting.

b. *Syrup* iodide of iron:

Iodine . . . . 1|5   23 gr.
Powdered iron . . . . 2|5   38 gr.
Syrup armoraciæ . . . . 1000|0   2 pts.

Two tablespoonfuls a day.

148. IODOFORM.

a. Iodoform . . . . 1|0   15 gr.
   Vaseline . . . . 10|0   2½ʒ

b. *Iodoform collodion:*

Iodoform . . . . 5|0   75 gr.
Flexible collodion . . . . 50|0   1ℨ 5ʒ

149. IODOL.

Inodorous; non-irritant. Takes the place of iodoform.

   a. As a *powder;* or,

   b. As an *ointment:*

Iodol . . . . 2|0		$\frac{1}{3}$
White vaseline . . . . } āā 8|0		$\frac{2}{3}$
Lanolin		

150. IODOPHENOCHLORAL.

Mixture of equal parts tincture of iodine, carbolic acid, and chloral.

Carefully touch up margin of lids in unyielding ulcerous blepharitis.

151. IRIDEREMIA.—ABSENCE OF THE IRIS.

Where there is photophobia: Smoked glasses, stenopæic glasses, circular tattooing of the cornea.

152. IRIDOCHOROIDITIS.—IRIDOCYCLO-CHOROIDITIS.

Acute stage: Mydriatics (233).—Antiphlogistic treatment (bloodletting at temple or mastoid process.—Dark room.—Avoid all congestions, alcohol, spiced meats, etc., as well as all food which is hard to digest.—Diaphoresis and diuresis (305).—Medicated foot-baths (118).

Chronic stage: Paracentesis of the anterior chamber. Iridectomy.—Massage of the eyeball.—Poultices (255) several hours daily.—Dark glasses.—Derivative treatment.

In case of syphilis: Specific treatment (291).

153. IRIS, ANGIOMA OF THE.

Excision where it irritates.

154. IRIS, COLOBOMA OF THE.

Where there is photophobia: Smoked glasses.
Tattooing of the cornea adapted in color to the iris.

155. IRIS, CYST OF THE.

As long as cysts do not give rise to inflammation: Wait; otherwise excision.

156. IRIS, CYSTICERCUS OF THE.

Excision (iridectomy) of the part of the iris containing the parasite.

Iris, Foreign Body of the. *See* under the heading of FOREIGN BODY OF THE CORNEA (84).

157. IRIS, GUMMATA OF THE.

Energetic specific treatment (291).

Iridectomy is indicated where gummata are few and very near to each other. It will always be made where synechiæ are present.

158. IRIS, SARCOMA OF THE.

Where tumor is very small and circumscribed and where the eye shows no sign of deeper trouble: Excision. Enucleation is safer.

159. IRIS, TRAUMA OF THE.

Foreign body of the iris: Simple extraction or iridectomy according to the case.

Prolapse of the iris: Excision or cauterization of the prolapsed part. Antiseptic dressing (101).

160. IRIS, TUBERCLE OF THE.

According to extent: Excision or enucleation.

Where patient shows symptoms of advanced tuberculosis of other organs: Symptomatic treatment.

161. IRITIS, Plastic, Rheumatic, Arthritic, Blennorrhœic, Syphilitic.

Mydriatics: Atropine (23 *a*), alternating with duboisine (102), or combined with cocaine (23 *b*), or a combination of atropine, cocaine, and duboisine (23 *c*).—Should the pupil not be enlarged by these solutions: Extract of belladonna or duboisine in substance (having care to close lachrymal points by pressure).—Close the eyes for at least five minutes after instillation.—Always watch the intra-ocular tension. As soon as tonus is $+$: Replace the mydriatics mentioned by scopolamine (284).

Rest for the eyes. Bandage the eye affected; dark room or smoked glasses according to cause and intensity of the disease.

Avoid sudden changes of temperature, draughts, etc.

Bloodletting or dry leeches at temple. Iodine ointment (146 *b*).—*Poultices* (255), hot compresses. For severe pain: Hypodermic injection of morphine (231 *c*).—Laxatives, diuresis, and diaphoresis (305).

IRITIS

Etiologic treatment: Where there are other symptoms of *rheumatism*, salicylate of soda (275), antipyrin (15), antifebrin (14), alkalies, acetate of potassium (254), lithia water (225 *b*).—Turkish baths.

In case of urethral *blennorrhœa*: Salol (278) and energetic treatment of the urethral trouble.

In *syphilis*: Specific treatment (291).

For dysmenorrhœa, scrofula, and anæmia: Strengthening treatment [arsenic (20), iron (164), etc.].

Continue mydriatics for some time after inflammatory symptoms have disappeared. Should synechiæ capable of bringing on relapses remain, iridectomy may be indicated.

162. IRITIS, SEROUS.

Treatment similar to that of interstitial keratitis (170).

General treatment: Tonics.—Diaphoresis (305), species sudorificæ (290), moist pack.

Local treatment: Atropine (23) (stop when tonus is +).—Hot compresses.—Poultices (255). Should deposits form on the posterior surface of the cornea: *Paracentesis. Withdraw* the needle *slowly*: thereupon open the wound by light pressure upon its edge with a spatula, so as to let the aqueous humor escape drop by drop. Repeat this on following days without renewing puncture.

In case of *relapse*: Change of climate, sojourn in the country.

163. IRITIS, TRAUMATIC.

The *only form of iritis in which iced compresses are indicated.* Otherwise about the same treatment as in ordinary iritis (161).

164. IRON.

a. *Sulphate* of iron . . . . 1|0 to 2|0   15 gr. to ½ʒ
   Distilled water . . . .   150|0   5ʒ
   Collyrium.

b. *Blaud's Pills:*
   Sulphate of iron . . . . } āā 15|0   āā ½ʒ
   Carbonate of potassium . . . . }
   Tragacanth . . . . } q. s. for 100 pills.
   Glycerin . . . . }
   3 to 5 pills a day.

c. Tincture of iron *malate.*
   Immediately after or during meals 5 to 10 drops in water.

d. *Ammonium citrate* with *iron pyrophosphate* . } equal parts.
   Sugar of milk . . . . }
   Twice daily according to age of child 1|0 *to* 3|0 *of the mixture in milk or soup.*

Wine of Iron and Quinine Citrate. *See* QUININE (259 *a*).

Syrup, Iodide of Iron. *See* IODINE (147 *b*).

Iron Baths. *See* MEDICINAL BATHS (25 *c*).

165. JEQUIRITY, MACERATION OF.

Macerate in one pint of water 10|0 (2½ʒ) of *old* shelled jequirity seeds for 24 hours.

166. JUNIPER OIL.

a. Pure juniper oil

Or better:
b. Juniper oil . . . . 2|0   ⅓
   Olive oil . . . . 3|0   45 gr.
   Apply to border of lids in blepharitis.

The oil penetrates into the eye easily and causes great irritation.

167. KEFIR.
a Weak kefir (has fermented 24 hours).
b. Medium strong kefir (has fermented 48 hours).
c. Strong kefir (has fermented 72 hours).

Take in small quantities at a time. Maximum: 3 quarts daily.

Keratitis of Stellwag. See DEEP PUNCTATED KERATITIS (174).

168. KERATITIS THROUGH LAGOPH-THALMUS.

Close lids by sutures, leaving an opening which permits cleaning of the eye with aseptic solutions. Where surgical interference is not permitted: Dry aseptic dressing during the night; repeated instillations of milk, glycerin, or mucilaginous fluids during the day. Pilocarpine (251 *a*) or eserine (111).

Keratitis, Eczematous. See PHLYCTENULAR KERATITIS (173).

Keratitis, Fascicular. See PHLYCTENULAR KERATITIS (173).

169. KERATITIS, FILAMENTOUS.

Hasten and facilitate the abnormal exfoliation of the epithelial layer by instillations of an aqueous solution of hydrochlorate of ammonia 2 : 100.

6 to 10 times a day.

170. KERATITIS, INTERSTITIAL.—PARENCHYMATOUS KERATITIS.

In the *beginning*: Atropine (23 a). Stop as soon as pupil is dilated.—Poultices (255), 4 to 10 hours a day.—Steam-douches (99 a).

For intense pain: Hot fomentations with

Extract of belladonna	3|0	45 gr.
Distilled water	200|0	6℥ 5₃

One tablespoonful in one-half pint of hot water (35° to 40° C.).

Later (when inflammatory symptoms are less pronounced) lessen hot applications slowly and add massage of the cornea, at first once, then twice, to three times daily for 2 to 5 minutes. Use for massage calomel ointment (33 a) or:

Lanolin . . . . } āā 1	0	āā 15 gr.
Blue ointment . . . . }		
Yellow vaseline 2	0	⅓

After massage bathe the open eyes with a boric acid solution (4 : 100) or a solution of biborate of soda (1 : 150).

To *hasten resorption* by vascularization: Instil rancid oil or touch up corneal limbus or conjunctival sac with the galvano-cautery.

General tonic treatment.—Rational and strengthening food.—Hygienic diet: Open air, exercise, medicated baths (25), iron (164), quinine (259), arsenic (20).—Sojourn in the country or at the sea-shore.

Where heredity is proved and child is not too weak: Energetic antisyphilitic treatment (291), interrupted every 2 to 3 weeks by 5 days of rest.

171. KERATITIS, NEUROPARALYTIC.—INDOLENT ULCER OF THE CORNEA.

Aseptic protective bandage.—Antiseptic washes.—Eserine (111) or pilocarpine (251 a). Galvanic current; positive pole held at neck, negative pole on closed lids.

172. KERATITIS, PANNOUS.—CORNEAL PANNUS. SUPERFICIAL VASCULAR KERATITIS.

Treat the *cause* [foreign bodies, chalky deposits, trichiasis (314) and distichiasis (97), entropion (106), granular conjunctivitis (75), etc.].

Eserine (111) or pilocarpine (251 a) if there are no symptoms of iritis.—Direct massage with finely powdered boric acid (30 c) (after cocainizing).—Yellow oxide ointment (10 : 100 !).—Insufflations of antipyrin powder and gentle massage [*intense reaction*]. Or:

Red oxide of mercury	0|15	2½ gr.
Camphor	0|10	1½ gr.
Vaseline . . . . } aa 1|0 to 3	00 aa 15 gr. to 45 gr.
Lanolin		

In *unyielding cases:* Abrasion of the region of the corneal limbus down to the sclera, followed by scarification of the sclera. Peritomy. Peridectomy, followed by scarification of the episcleral tissue.

Keratitis, Parenchymatous. *See* INTERSTITIAL KERATITIS (170).

173. KERATITIS, PHLYCTENULAR, ECZEMATOUS.—ECZEMA OF THE CORNEA.—FASCICULAR KERATITIS.

Forbid bandage.—Smoked glasses.—Myotics (235) [atropine (23 *a*) only in cases of threatening iritis; combine it with cocaine (23 *b*) where there is blepharospasm].—Massage with calomel (33 *c*) [forbid internal use of iodine preparations].

Several times daily compresses with sublimate ($\frac{1}{5}$ to $\frac{1}{2}$ in 1000) or with boric acid (4 : 100).

In case of small *superficial ulcerations:* Replace calomel powder by iodol (149), aristol (18 *a*), calomel (33 *c*), or yellow oxide (229 *a*) ointment.

Where ulcers are deep and large : Treatment of ulcerous keratitis (176).

Should the phlyctenulæ *not yield to calomel:* Cauterize either with point of a mitigated nitrate of silver pencil (287 *b*, *β*) or with galvano-cautery, followed by a well-fitting bandage moistened with sublimate (1 : 3000) or with the following solution :

Neutral sulphate of eserine	0|20	3 gr.
Boric acid	2|00	30 gr.
Glycerin	40|00	1ℨ 2½ℨ
Distilled water	10|00	2½ℨ

For *photophobia* and *blepharospasm :* Dip the face in fresh water, whereupon rub vigorously with a rough towel ; let the child walk or run in a room in which obstacles have been placed so as to force it to open its eyes.—In unyielding cases : Open the lids by force and keep them open during from 5 to 15 minutes.—Blepharorrhaphy.

Attend to the *eczema* and *acne* of the face and head: Soap the head vigorously with tar soap and make appropriate applications with ointments. See ECZEMA OF THE LIDS (197).

Attend to the scrofulous rhinitis: Clean nasal cavities frequently. Nasal douches (100). Insufflations of:

Subnitrate of bismuth	20|0	5ʒ
Tannin	4|0	1ʒ
Powdered benzoin	10|0	2½ʒ

General antiscrofulous treatment: Baths with bran (25 *a*) or sea-salt (25 *d*); cod-liver oil (54); iron preparations (164), arsenic (20), syrupus armoraciæ (308); kola (179). Sojourn in country or at seashore [avoid sandy beaches].

Combat *swelling* of the *conjunctiva* by cauterization with the pure (287 *b*) or mitigated (287 *b*, *a*) nitrate of silver pencil.

For *pain:* Collyrium (52 *a*) or ointment (52 *b*) with cocaine or morphine (231).

Cauterize fissures brought on by tears with the nitrate of silver pencil (287 *b*) and apply the following ointment:

Acetate of lead	2|00	½ʒ
Extract of opium	0|10	1½ gr.
Balsam of Peru	5|00	1½ʒ
Fresh lard	30|00	1ʒ

174. KERATITIS, DEEP PUNCTATED.—KERATITIS OF STELLWAG.

[*Do not confound with the deposits on posterior surface of cornea through serous iritis.*]

In the *beginning*: Atropine (23 *a*) and energetic antiphlogistic treatment.

Later: Eserine (111) or pilocarpine (251 *a*). Yellow oxide ointment (229 *b*). Poultices (255); hot fomentations with an infusion of chamomile flowers or belladonna leaves. Hypodermic injections of pilocarpine (305 *b*). Systemic treatment of arthritis and gout: Lithium salicylate (225 *a*).

175. KERATITIS, SUPERFICIAL NON-VASCULAR.

Atropine (23 *a*), where there are symptoms of impending iritis; otherwise, eserine (111) or pilocarpine (251 *a*).—Poultices or hot compresses with boric acid (4 : 100).—Calomel (33 *a*), boric acid (30 *d*), or yellow oxide (229 *b*) ointments.

Keratitis, Superficial Vascular. *See* PANNOUS KERATITIS (172).

176. KERATITIS, ULCEROUS.—ULCER OF THE CORNEA.

Strict antisepsis.—Avoid cold applications.

Etiologic treatment: Foreign bodies, purulent conjunctivitis (69, 77), trachoma (75), dacryocystitis (91, 92) [in this last case the radical operation with scraping or cauterization of the lachrymal sac is the safest], ozaena: Repeated douches with sublimate (1 : 2000) and inhalations of:

Carbolic acid	5|0	75 gr.
Absolute alcohol	15|0	1 ʒ
Aqua ammonia	5|0	75 gr.
Distilled water	10|0	2½ ʒ

Bismuth, finely pulverized, to be used as a snuff every three hours.

KERATITIS

Antiseptic dressing (101) and hot compresses with sublimate (1 : 5000).—Apply chlorine water or chloride of zinc (325 c) with a brush.—Fomentations with salicylic acid (1 to 2 per 100).

Where fundus and sides of ulcer are *infiltrated*: Galvano-cauterization followed by free and prolonged irrigation with strong antiseptic solutions, or : scraping with sharp spoon followed by the application of a strong sublimate solution (1 : 500), or : subconjunctival injection of a sublimate solution (1 : 2000) [*daily amount one syringe of Pravaz*].

Instillations of atropine (23 a) where perforation is not to be feared.

Where perforation is to be feared from lack of resistance of the ulcerated cornea : Myotics (235).

As soon as *perforation* seems *inevitable :* Perform it carefully with the galvano-cautery. Previously instil atropine (23 a) where ulcer is central, or a myotic (235) where ulcer is peripheral.

In case of *ulcus rodens with hypopyon :* Keratotomy, passing through the centre of the ulcer, or paracentesis from below parallel to corneal margin, followed by washing of the anterior chamber with :

Salicylate of eserine	0|12	2 gr.
Boric acid	1|00	15 gr.
Distilled water	25|00	6½ℨ

Thereupon instil :

Neutral sulphate of atropine	0|50	8 gr.
Neutral sulphate of quinine	20|00	5ℨ
Sterilized distilled water	30|00	1ℨ

Then : Antiseptic dressing (101).

Should *pain* caused by the ulcer be very great :

Morphine injections (231 c) at temple, instillations of cocaine (52 a), or fomentations and compresses with:

Chlorine water . . . . } āā	200|0	āā 6ʒ 6ʒ
Lime water		
Hydrochlorate of cocaine	4|0	1ʒ
and three times a day an instillation of 3 drops of:		
Extract of Calabar bean	0|30	4½ gr.
Pure glycerin	10|00	2½ʒ

For *deep indolent ulcer* of the cornea, the treatment is the same as that of neuroparalytic keratitis (171).

177. KERATOCONUS.

Stenopæic glasses.—Spherical, conical, or torical glasses placed before the cornea or in contact with it.

Where necessary: Galvano-cautery applied to apex of keratoconus, followed by aseptic pressure bandage.—Ablation of the apex or a segment of the cornea.

178. KERATOGLOBUS.

In the *beginning:* Pressure bandage.—Myotics (235).—Peripheral iridectomy.—Section through the ciliary muscle.—Sclerotomy.—Repeated paracentesis.

Where the prominence of the keratoglobus hinders the movements of the lids: Ablation of the prominent part or enucleation.

179. KOLA.

a. Kola wine.
  50|0 to 100|0 (1½ʒ to 3ʒ) a day.

b. Fluid extract of kola.
  10 drops several times a day.

Lachrymal Sac, Blennorrhœa of the. *See* PURULENT DACRYOCYSTITIS (92).

Lachrymal Sac, Fistula of the. *See* under the heading of CHRONIC DACRYOCYSTITIS (91).

180. LACHRYMAL PASSAGES, OBSTRUCTION OF THE.

Methodical *use of probes* without slitting lachrymal canals except where absolutely necessary. The *ends* of the probes should be *olive-shaped.*—At each dilatation leave them in place for about 15 minutes.—*Do not probe more often than necessary,* just often enough to keep passages open for tears and injections.—Medicines should be injected with a *syringe,* the *point* of which is *also olive-shaped.*

In *unyielding cases:* Ablation of the palpebral or orbital lachrymal gland [operating from conjunctival side] or :

Electrolysis of the lachrymal passages : A Bowman probe (insulated with the exception of the end) is introduced into the duct [avoid splitting canaliculus, if possible ; where this is unavoidable it must be done some time before this process is tried]. Connect probe with the negative pole. The positive pole wrapped in a little moist cotton is placed in the nostril of the same side.—Increase intensity of current by the aid of the rheostat slowly up to a maximum of 5 milliamperes. If a strong current is used, we have to fear the formation of scars.—The application should last no longer than five minutes in all.—*Decrease* the strength of the current to zero *very gradually*.—The operation can be repeated several times at an interval of a few days.—The batteries are the same as those used for the continuous current. They should give a 40-milliampere current at least.—Milliamperemeter and rheostat are indispensable.—The procedure is used particularly in cases of inflammatory origin.

Where there is *suppuration*: Slit the *upper* lachrymal canal and treat as chronic dacryocystitis (91).

181. LACHRYMAL POINTS, EVERSION OF THE.

Where palpebral tissue has undergone no change bring the points back into their normal position by making a channel, the posterior wall of which is excised or cauterized.

Special treatment is necessary where the eversion is caused by conjunctival or palpebral trouble.

182. LACTIC ACID.

Lactic acid	1|0 to	3|0	15 gr. to 45 gr.
Distilled water		100|0	3℥ 8℥

183. LACTOPHENIN.

0|50 to 1|0 (8 gr. to 15 gr.) before retiring.

Lagophthalmus. *See* PARALYSIS OF THE ORBICULAR MUSCLE (244), and KERATITIS THROUGH LAGOPHTHALMUS (168).

184. LANOLIN.

Excellent excipient for ointments ; active of itself in light forms of blepharitis. Its consistence is but little modified by temperature. It is well to add a more oily body to it, for instance : Vaseline (30|0 to 40|0 to 100|0 of lanolin). Use also :

Pure lanolin	65|0	2₃
Liquid paraffin	30|0	1₃
Ceresin	5|0	1½₃

185. LEAD.

a.
Subacetate of lead	00|50	8 gr.
Rose water	30|00	1₃
Distilled water	120|00	4₃

b.
Subacetate of lead	0|50 to 2|0	½₃
Distilled water	8|0	2₃
White vaseline	10|0	2½₃
Pure lanolin	10|0	2½₃

Apply on closed lids

c.
Subacetate of lead	00|25	4 gr.
Distilled water	8|00	2₃
White vaseline	10|00	2½₃
Pure lanolin	10|00	2½₃

Apply to conjunctiva of lids.

d. Compresses of subacetate of lead solution.

20 drops of liquor plumbi subacetici in a bowl containing about 400|0 (13₃) of lukewarm water ; steep pledgets of hygroscopic cotton into this solution and apply twice or more times daily on the eyes during from a half to one hour ; renew pledgets every 3 minutes.

186. LEECHES, APPLICATION OF.

According to the disease and state of general health of patients : Apply 2, 3, or 4 leeches, and let the blood flow as long as desirable, according to the case.—Take a tube or vial narrow enough to permit of placing the leech just at the spot you wish. *Clean* this spot *beforehand.*—Should *leeches refuse* to suck : Pour 2 or 3 drops of white wine or some drops of diluted vinegar into the glass which holds them.—Usually leeches are left until they drop off.

To *keep up* the *bleeding :* Apply a linseed poultice.

To *stop bleeding :* Apply a piece of tinder or hæmostatic cotton upon the incision made by the leech and dust with powdered alum.

Where necessary : Tight pressure bandage.

187. LETTUCE, DISTILLED WATER OF LEAVES OF.

For soothing compresses. Can be added to the different collyria.

188. LIDS, ABSCESS OF THE.

Etiologic treatment.—Poultices (255).—Incision parallel to the free margin.—Drainage.—Compresses with sublimate (1 : from 2000 to 5000).

Lids, Angioma of the. *See* ERECTILE TUMORS OF THE LIDS (217).

189. LIDS, ANTHRAX OF THE.

Incision in the shape of a cross, thereupon alternately poultices (255) and sublimate compresses (1 : 500).—Strengthening food.—Tonics.

190. LIDS, BITES OF INSECTS ON.

Iced compresses.—Repeated applications of ammonia mixed with ether or chloroform (10 a).

191. LIDS, BLACK HEADS OF THE.
Expression.

192. LIDS, BURNS OF THE.

a. Slight burns (burns of *first degree*, causing rubefaction only).

Finely powdered bismuth.—Linimentum calcis (223).

or:

Hydrochlorate of cocaine	3|0	45 gr.
Vaseline . . . . } āā	20|0	āā 5ʒ
Distilled water		
Lanolin	5|0	75 gr.

b. More severe burns (burns of *second degree*, causing vesiculation).

Hydrochlorate of cocaine	1|50	23 gr.
Salol	3|00	45 gr.
Vaseline	25|00	6½ʒ

or:

Aristol ointment (18 *b, c*).

or:

Iodoform	4|00	1ʒ
Extract of conium leaves	2|00	½ʒ
Carbolic acid	0|05	1 gr.
Unguentum rosatum	30|00	1ʒ

Before applying any of these three ointments open the vesicles and wash carefully.

c. Severe burns (burns of the *third degree* with destruction of tissue).

Europhen	3|0	45 gr.
Olive oil	7|0	2ʒ
Vaseline	60|0	2ʒ
Lanolin	30|0	1ʒ

Renew this application but every third or fourth day.

193. LIDS, CHROMIDROSIS OF THE.

Oleaginous inunctions.—Etiologic treatment (dysmenorrhœa).

194. LIDS, COLOBOMA OF THE.

Freshen up the edges and unite carefully by numerous sutures.

Lids, Cyst of the. *See* HYDATID OF THE LIDS (205).

195. LIDS, CYSTICERCUS OF THE.
Excision.

196. LIDS, ECCHYMOSIS OF THE.

Pressure bandage.—Compresses with subacetate of lead solution (185 *d*).—Fomentations with :

Tincture of arnica	2|0	ʒss
Water	80|0	2ʒ 5ʒ

197. LIDS, ECZEMA AND ACNE OF THE LIDS AND NEIGHBORING PARTS.

Systemic treatment of the *scrofulous diathesis:* Arsenic (20), iron (164), cod-liver oil (54), baths with bran (25 *a*), and sea-salt (25 *d*).

Forbid taking of *too much food, abuse of meat and spices.* Total *abstinence from wine and alcohol.*—Keep bowels loose.

Minute Cleanliness.—Wash head with tar soap, pluck out lashes and hairs which are about to fall out; acne pustules or pimples to be incised and squeezed out.

Prophylaxis.—Wash repeatedly with 50 per cent. alcohol, to dissolve sebaceous masses obstructing the canaliculi of the glands, having care that the alcohol does not penetrate into conjunctival sac.

Antiseptic Treatment.—Repeated compresses with sublimate (from 1 : 800 to 1 : 500).

Ointments with boric acid (30 *d*), ichthyol (139), naphtol (236 *b*), tannin (310 *b*), calomel (33 *b*), sulphur (304), gallanol (120), ointment of Hebra (130) or Pagenstecher (229).

Let the ointment remain on the lid several hours, then wipe off carefully and dust with an inert powder: Rice powder, talc, or brush the lid with:

Oxide of zinc	50|0	1ʒ 5ʒ
Salicylic acid	5|0	75 gr.
Starch }	āā 2|0	āā ½ʒ
Glycerin		
Water	75|0	2½ʒ

In *unyielding cases* use one of the following ointments:

Naphtol	10|0	2½ʒ
Precipitated sulphur	50|0	1ʒ 5ʒ
Tar soap }	āā 20|0	āā 5ʒ
Vaseline		

Application to remain on lids from 30 minutes to 1 hour, whereupon wash with hot water.

LIDS

Resorcin . . . . } āā 0|50 to 1|0	āā 8 gr. to 15 gr.
Salicylic acid	
Oxide of zinc	2|0	½ 𝔷
Vaseline	18|0	4½ 𝔷

This ointment will not decompose; it may therefore be applied at night and replaced in the morning by cold cream or rice powder.

Subnitrate of bismuth . . . . 10|0	2½ 𝔷
Oxide of zinc . . . . 2|0	½ 𝔷
Glycerin . . . . 8|0	2 𝔷
Carbolic acid . . . . 20 drops.|0	20 gtt.
White vaseline . . . . 30|0	1 𝔷

3 times daily during one-half hour.

Naphtol . . . . 10|0	2½ 𝔷
Camphor . . . . 1|0	15 gr.
White vaseline . . . . 90|0	3 𝔷

During 15 minutes. Soothe any stronger irritation following by an oil or an emollient paste.

Between each application of any of these ointments, dust diseased parts with an inert powder.

Lotions:

Tincture of male fern . . . . 30|0	1 𝔷
Absolute alcohol . . . . 15|0	½ 𝔷
Tincture of myrrh . . . . 4|0	1 𝔷
Crude powdered opium . . . . 4|0	1 𝔷

Shake before using Brush the diseased parts carefully twice a day with this solution and wash rigorously with an alkaline soap afterwards.

Precipitated sulphur . . . . 1|0	15 gr.
Spirits of camphor . . . . 5|0	75 gr.
Lime water . . . . 80|0	2 𝔷 5 𝔷

Tumenol	5.0	75 gr.
Sulphuric ether	} āā 15.0	āā 1₃
Absolute alcohol		
Glycerin or distilled water	30.0	1₃
Finely powdered iodoform	10.00	2½₃
Pure cocaine	0.30	5 gr.
Mix with care and add:		
Menthol	0.50	8 gr.
Spirits of lavender	20.00	5₃

The use of these numerous therapeutic means must vary and adapt itself to the different forms of eczema.

Should the disease *persist*: Carefully cauterize with galvano-cautery or apply a mixture of equal parts of:

> Tincture of iodine,
> Pure carbolic acid,
> Chloral.

In both cases use a non-irritating ointment after the applications.

198. LIDS, EMPHYSEMA OF THE.

Etiologic treatment.—Pressure.—Massage.

Lids, Epithelioma of the. *See* MALIGNANT TUMORS OF THE LIDS (218).

199. LIDS, ERYSIPELAS OF THE.

Systemic treatment.—Purgatives.—Antipyretics.

Energetic local treatment. [*Danger of infiltration of the orbit* on account of the laxity of tissue, and if progressive, of *meningitis* by immigration of streptococci passing through the veins of Santorini.]—Try to *limit* the erysipelas to the face by:

Injections of sublimate (*1 : 1000, several syringefuls*), compresses with carbolic acid (3 : 100) or sublimate (1 : 1000); repeated energetic washes with alcohol (90 : 100).—Brush with tincture of iodine (147 *a*). *From the beginning lids should be closed* by adhesive plaster and any fatty substance.

According to extent, seat, and intensity : Ice, inunctions with double mercurial ointment (291 *b*).— Friction with ichthyol (10 : 100) or with :

Traumatacin	120|00	4ʒ
Resorcin	1|50	23 gr.

or with :

Carbolic acid . . . . } āā	15|0	āā 1ʒ
Alcohol		
Spirits of turpentine	30|0	1ʒ
Glycerin	50|0	1ʒ 5ʒ

Shake this mixture before using.

or apply :

Flexible collodion	20|0	5ʒ
Iodoform	1|0	15 gr.

or :

Flexible collodion	30|0	1ʒ
Sublimate	1|0	15 gr.

During intervals dust with an inert powder, such as : Talc, starch, rice.

Where there is *great pain:* Linimentum calcis (223).

200. LIDS, FAVUS OF THE.

Pluck out all the eyelashes and even the hairs of the eyebrows.—Vigorous washes with tar soap, followed by friction with sublimate (1 : 400).

201. LIDS, FIBROMA OF THE.

Excision, followed where necessary by a plastic operation.

Lids, Furuncle of the. *See* STYE (301).

202. LIDS, FURUNCULOSIS OF THE.

Open air.—Bodily exercise.—Regulate stools.—Local treatment similar to that of blepharitis (26, 27).

Wash regularly with:

Salicylic acid	5|0	75 gr.
Biborate of soda	3|0	45 gr.
Distilled water	500|0	1 pt.

or with:

Precipitated sulphur	3|0	45 gr.
Hydrochlorate of ammonium	1|0	15 gr.
Rose water	50|0	1ʒ 5ʒ
Spirits of camphor	10|0	2½ʒ

Shake solution before using.

In *unyielding cases* apply every evening on lids and between lashes:

Spirits of camphor	1|00	15 gr.
Precipitated sulphur	1|00	15 gr.
Lime water } āā	10|00 āā	2½ʒ
Rose water		
Gum arabic	0|20	3 gr.

Shake solution before using.

203. LIDS, HERPES FEBRILIS OF THE.

Inert powder: Talc, rice powder.—Where itching is great: Ointment with cocaine (52 *b*).

204. LIDS, HERPES ZOSTER OF THE.

Starch, talc, ointment with cocaine (52 b) or morphine (231 b).—Liniment with chloroform (41 b), *having care that liniment does not penetrate into cul-de-sac.*

Galvanic current for periorbital neuralgia.—Compresses with:

Corrosive sublimate	0|15	2½ gr.
Hydrochlorate of cocaine	2|50	40 gr.
Distilled water	100|00	3℥ 2ℨ

Systemic treatment: Antifebrin (14), antipyrin (15 a), salicylate of soda (275).

In cases in which *cornea* and *conjunctiva* are *affected:* Treat according to rules set down under the heading of Herpes of the Cornea (85) and Zona Ophthalmica (326).

205. LIDS, HYDATID OF THE.

Excision of part of the wall of the cyst.

206. LIDS, HYPERÆMIA OF.

Hygienic treatment.—Open air.—Compresses with subacetate of lead solution (185 d) or with non-irritant collyrium (29, 30 a, 185 a).—Regulate stools.

207. LIDS, IMPETIGO OF.

Systemic treatment: Cod-liver oil (54), iodides (147 b), iron preparations (164), alkalies, arsenic (20).

During *inflammatory stage* apply the following ointment as a plaster on a thin piece of linen:

Boric acid	1|0	15 gr.
Emplastrum hydrargyri compos.	5|0	75 gr.
Vaseline	30|0	1 ʒ

As soon as every trace of inflammation has disappeared:

Simple lead plaster	20|00	5 ʒ
Oxide of red lead	2|50	38 gr.
Red sulphide of mercury	1|00	15 gr.

Renew every day, washing with a solution of spirits of camphor before each dressing.

208. LIDS, LIPOMA OF THE.

Excision, followed where necessary by a plastic operation.

209. LIDS, LUPUS OF THE.

Energetic scraping with the sharp spoon.—Excision.—Cauterize wound with thermo-cautery.—Plastic operation when lupus is cured.

Lids, Melanosarcoma of the. *See* MALIGNANT TUMORS OF THE LIDS (218).

210. LIDS, MILIUM OF THE.

Incision.—Expression.—Cauterization.

211. LIDS, MOLLUSCUM CONTAGIOSUM OF THE.

Total extraction or ablation where tumor is pediculated.

Lids, Molluscum Lipomatoides of the. *See* XANTHELASMA OF THE LIDS (222).

212. LIDS, ŒDEMA OF THE.

Treat the cause.—Locally: Compresses with subacetate of lead solution (185 *d*).

In unyielding cases: Apply flexible collodion, or brush with:

Spirits of lavender . . . . } āā 20	0	āā 53
Spirits of rosemary		
Oil of lemon 2	0	15

Scarifications where other measures fail.

213. LIDS, PAPILLOMA OF THE.

Ligature.—Ablation.—Cauterization with chemicals or the thermo-cautery.

Lids, Phlegmon of the. *See* ABSCESS OF THE LIDS (188).

214. LIDS, PHTHIRIASIS OF THE.

Energetic washes with tar soap.—*Careful* application of mercurial ointment.

Lids, Sarcoma of the. *See* MALIGNANT TUMORS OF THE LIDS (218).

215. LIDS, SEBORRHŒA OF THE.

1. *Seborrhœa sicca.*

Remove the pellicles and scales hindering the regular drainage of the product of the sebaceous glands several times a day. Facilitate this cleaning by a previous application of some non-irritant ointment.—*See* BLEPHARITIS (26).

2. *Seborrhœa oleosa.*

Systemic treatment. [Often Dysmenorrhœa.]— Minute cleanliness.

Dry the lids several times a day with tissue-paper and brush with:

Precipitated sulphur	1|0	15 gr.
Linseed oil	5|0	75 gr.

Cold (98 *a*) or Scottish (98 *b*) douches upon the nape of the neck and the vertebral column.—Wash the lids with water to which some alcohol has been added, or with cologne water.

Careful applications with juniper oil mixed with some alcohol or mitigated by olive oil (166 *b*), or with spirits of alkaline soap.

216. LIDS, TELANGIECTASIS OF THE.

Repeated punctures with the galvano-cautery.— Excision, followed where necessary by a plastic operation.

217. LIDS, ERECTILE TUMORS OF THE.
Ablation.

218. LIDS, MALIGNANT TUMORS OF THE.

[Epithelioma, Sarcoma, Melanosarcoma.]

Radical ablation, followed by a plastic operation. —*Save the smallest pieces of healthy palpebral tissue,* on account of its vitality and the difficulty found to replace it.

219. LIDS, TYLOSIS OF THE.

Energetic massage upon a shell or horn plate during ½ to 1 hour with:

White precipitate of mercury	0|05 to 0|1	1 gr. to 2 gr.
Cold cream	5|0	75 gr.

220. LIDS, ULCERS OF THE, through Syphilis or Smallpox.

According to case: Antisyphilitic treatment (291) or cauterization.—Iodol (149 *b*) or aristol ointment (18 *b, c*).

Lids, Warts of the. *See* PAPILLOMA OF THE LIDS (213).

221. LIDS, WOUNDS OF THE.

Unite the edges of wound by suture *as exactly as possible.*—Antiseptic pressure bandage (101).

222. LIDS, XANTHELASMA OF THE.—XANTHOMA.

Where tumor is *small:* Cauterization with nitric or hydrochloric acid.

Where it is *large:* Multiple ligatures.—Coagulating injection [insulate diseased part by pressure]. —Excision followed by a plastic operation.

Lids, Xanthoma of the. *See* XANTHELASMA OF THE LIDS (222).

223. LINIMENTUM CALCIS.

Lime water	} āā 100|00	āā 3ʒ 2ʒ
Linseed oil or olive oil		
Thymol	0|20	3 gr.

Apply to parts affected.

Linseed oil should have the preference in spite of its disagreeable odor.

224. LINIMENTS, SOOTHING.

a. Oil of sweet almond		60|0	2ʒ
Chloroform	30|0 to 40|0		1ʒ to 1ʒ 2½ʒ

b. Oil of hyoscyamus	100|0	3ʒ 2ʒ
Fluid extract belladonna	15|0	½ʒ
Tincture of opium	10|0	2½ʒ

Linseed Meal. *See* POULTICES (255).

225. LITHIUM.

a. Salicylate of lithium } āā 1|0 āā 15 gr.
   Sugar of milk

  One powder. To be taken in a half wineglassful of carbonated water. Four powders a day.

b. Lithia water.

Carbonate of lithium	1|0	15 gr.
Carbonated water	1000|0	2 pts.

  To be taken in two days.

226. LOSS OF THE EYELASHES.

Gallic acid	0|50	8 gr.
Oil of lavender	4 drops.	4 gtt.
Castor oil	2|00	½ʒ
Vaseline	5|00	1½ʒ

Lunar Caustic. *See* NITRATE OF SILVER (287 b).

Malt. *See* EXTRACT OF MALT (115).

227. MEMBRANE, PERSISTING PUPILLARY.

Where membrane is very thick: Iridectomy.— Otherwise refrain from any interference.

228. MENTHOL.

a. Menthol .... 0|75   12 gr.
    Hydrochlorate of cocaine .... 0|25   4 gr.
    Chloral hydrate .... 0|15   2½ gr.
    Vaseline .... 5|00   1⅓ ℨ

It is also used in the form of:

b. Pencils.
    For local applications.

229. MERCURY.

Pagenstecher's Ointment = Yellow Oxide Ointment.

a. Yellow oxide of mercury .. 0|20 to 0|50   3 gr. to 8 gr.
    White vaseline .... 10|00   2⅓ ℨ

    Apply to border of lids in the morning; wipe off carefully after one hour.

b. Yellow oxide of mercury .. 0|10 to 0|20   1½ gr. to 3 gr.
    White vaseline .... 10|00   2⅓ ℨ

    Triturate thoroughly before mixing and add vaseline gradually. Introduce into cul-de-sac.— Where ointment irritates: Add 0|1 to 0|2 of poplar-tree charcoal (36) to it.

Red Oxide Ointment.

c. Red oxide of mercury .... 0|10 to 0|20   1½ gr. to 3 gr.
    White vaseline ...... 10|00   2⅓ ℨ
    To be used as above.

White Precipitate Ointment.

d. White precipitate of mercury .... 0|50   8 gr.
    White vaseline .... 10|00   2⅓ ℨ
    Apply to border of lids.

20 drops of the tincture of benzoin can be added to these ointments, or the simple vaseline can be replaced by benzoinated vaseline [*made with gum, not with tincture*].

MERCURY

e. Salicylate of mercury . . . . 0|40   6 gr.
   Tincture of opium . . . . 10 drops.   10 gtt.
   Extract of gentian, q. s.
     For 20 pills; 2 to 3 pills a day.

f. Protoiodide of mercury . . . . 1|00   15 gr.
   Powdered opium . . . . 0|30   5 gr.
   Extract of liquorice and liquorice powder, q. s.
     For 50 pills; 2 pills three times a day.

g. Tannate of mercury . . . . 3|0   45 gr.
   Extract of liquorice and liquorice powder, q. s.
     For 60 pills; 1 to 2 pills three times a day.

All these pills are taken with or after meals.

h. Oxicyanide of mercury . . . . 1|0   15 gr.
   Distilled water . . . . 100|0 $3\frac{1}{4}$ ℥
    Solution for sterilizing instruments.

i. Biniodide of mercury . . . . 4|0   1 ℥
   Sterilized olive oil . . . . 1000|0   2 pts.

---

k. Biniodide of mercury . . . . 0|10 $1\frac{1}{2}$ gr.
   Iodide of potassium . . . . 5|00 $1\frac{1}{3}$ ℥
   Distilled water . . . . 5|00 $1\frac{1}{3}$ ℥
   Simple syrup . . . . 240|00   8 ℥
    2 tablespoonfuls a day for adults. *For children from 4 to 6 years:* a teaspoonful three times a day; *for the new-born:* half a teaspoonful twice daily.

l. Cyanide of mercury . . . . 0|20   3 gr.
   Distilled water . . . . 20|00   5 ℥
    One syringe = 0|01 ($\frac{1}{6}$ gr.) *cyanide of mercury.—Begin by injecting half a syringeful, and only in exceptional cases inject the maximum of 2 syringefuls* (0|02 = $\frac{1}{3}$ gr.).—*Every other day.*

The *cyanide of mercury* does *not coagulate albumen* and *remains soluble* in the tissues.

m. Benzoate of mercury	0|20	3 gr.
Chloride of sodium	0|20	3 gr.
Hydrochlorate of cocaine	0|05	1 gr.
Distilled water	20|00	5ʒ

Daily dose: one (Pravaz) syringeful.

n. Peptone	} āā	0|30	āā 5 gr.
Pure chloride of ammonia			
Corrosive sublimate		0|20	3 gr.
Glycerin		5|00	1½ʒ
Distilled water		15|00	½ʒ

Daily dose: one (Pravaz) syringeful.

Bichloride of Mercury and Peptonate of Mercury. *See* SUBLIMATE (302).

Mild Chloride of Mercury. *See* CALOMEL (33).

Simple Mercurial Ointment. *See* MERCURIAL INUNCTIONS (143).—**Double Mercurial Ointment.** *See* SPECIFIC TREATMENT (291 *b*).

Methylacetanilid. *See* EXALGIN (114).

230. METHYL, IODIDE OF.

Local application as a vesicant in neuralgia.

231. MORPHINE.

a. Hydrochlorate of morphine	0|30	5 gr.
White vaseline	6|00	1½ʒ

Introduce under the lids in cases of corneal ulcerations with violent pains.

b. Hydrochlorate of morphine	2|0	½ʒ
Benzoinated lard	30|0	1ʒ

Soothing ointment.

c. Hydrochlorate of morphine	0|10	1½ gr.
Spirits of peppermint	1|00	15 gr.
Distilled peppermint water	10|00	2⅔ ʒ

One syringe = 0|01 of morphine.

This solution is less subject to changes than those generally in use, still it is *better* to *dissolve* 0|01 (⅙ gr.) of the hydrochlorate of morphine in one cubic centimetre of sterilized water *immediately before injection*.

In case of *morphine poisoning:* Hypodermic injection of 0|001 ($\frac{1}{60}$ gr.) of the neutral sulphate of atropine [$\frac{2}{10}$ of a (Pravaz) syringeful of the ordinary collyrium (23 *a*)].—Where necessary, a second injection can be made at the end of 15 minutes, and even a third one after 30 minutes.

Inhalations of amyl nitrite (11).

Internally: Strong coffee, brandy, volatile salt (10 *b*).

Artificial respiration, massage, and friction of the body.

Muriatic Acid. *See* FOOT-BATHS (118).

232. MUSCÆ VOLITANTES.

Are often without signification: often due to overwork or some change of the deeper structures of the eye.

Rest.—Glasses correcting astigmatism and relieving accommodation.—In the bright light: Blue or smoked glasses.—In case of exudations in the vitreous, *see* CHOROIDITIS (47), RETINITIS (271).

Muscarin. *See* MYOTICS (235).

Mustard. *See* MEDICATED FOOT-BATHS (118) and SINAPISMS (288).

Mustard Paper. *See* SINAPISMS (288).

Mustard Plaster. *See* SINAPISMS (288).

233. MYDRIATICS.

[Dose and directions for use, *see* ATROPINE (23), HOMATROPINE (133), DUBOISINE (102), SCOPOLAMIN (284), COCAINE (52), and INSTILLATIONS OF COLLYRIA (141)].

They are *poisonous.*—*Dilate* the *pupil.*—*Increase intraocular tension* [scopolamin is perhaps the only exception].—*Paralyze* the *accommodation.*

For aseptic or antiseptic purposes 1|0 to 2|0 (15 gr. to ⅓) of a 1 : 1000 sublimate solution can be added to 10|0 of collyrium.

To obtain the *greatest possible effect*, the *pure salt* can be introduced, care being taken to compress the lachrymal passages so as to avoid poisonous effects.

In *small children* it is best to prescribe mydriatics in the form of an *ointment.*

a. *Atropine* (23). Mydriatic the most in use.—Very powerful.—Very poisonous.—Mydriasis lasts long.—Sometimes not tolerated by conjunctiva.

b. *Homatropine* (133). Action is more prompt but weaker.—Less poisonous.—Shorter mydriasis.

c. *Duboisine* (102). Is used where conjunctiva will not tolerate atropine, alone or also in combination with atropine and cocaine.

d. *Scopolamin* (284). Prompt and energetic action.—Limited duration of the paralysis of accommodation.—Very little poisonous.—Hardly increases intraocular tension.

It is indicated particularly where a tendency to an increased tension exists in cases of short duration and for determining refraction.

e. Cocaine (52). Very weak mydriatic action.—Adds to the effect when given in combination with other mydriatics.

f. Hyoscine and *hyoscyamine* have been abandoned on account of their uncertain action.

234. MYOPIA.

Patient hardly ever tolerates permanently the glass completely correcting his myopia; that is, the glass which gives him the best vision in the distance. A *weaker glass* giving him sufficient vision for distance is therefore *to be preferred*.

It is *nearly always better* for a myope to use *no concave glasses for near vision*. Myopia of a slight degree can even require convex glasses, particularly in myopes of mature age.—Where work demands a *distance beyond* that of the *far point* of the myope he should use the glass representing the difference between his myopia and the denominator of the working distance. For instance, let working distance be 50 cm. $= \frac{1}{2} m$, the denominator, that is, the corresponding refraction, is equal to 2 D. A myope of 5 D will receive No. $5-2 = 3$ D to see at this distance; a myope of 7 D, the concave glass $7-2 = 5$ D.

Myopes of a *very high degree* generally prefer to

use one eye alone for near work, renouncing binocular vision, whereby they have the advantage of *larger retinal images*.—The physician should recommend that patient does not get nearer to his work than the distance corresponding to the glass prescribed.

Prophylaxis and *hygiene of myopes:* From *early childhood* avoid fatiguing the eyes, even in the choice of playthings.—Moderate reading, good light, daylight by preference.—Good print. large letters, black on a white background, short lines.— Keep as far away as possible from object at which you look.—Avoid bending head forward too far. —Lean against back of chair in reading, write upon an inclined plane.—Light in reading should come from behind; from the left side and from above in writing.—Interrupt work frequently.—Avoid congestions to the head [constipation. excesses at meals, cold feet, tight clothing, sitting close to the lamp, etc.].—Room should be well ventilated, and work never be taken up immediately after a meal.

Strengthen the general health, exercise in the open air, gymnastic exercises.—Rest for the eyes, sojourn in the country.

Compare also Spasm of the Accommodation (2) and Sclero-choroiditis (47).

235. MYOTICS.

[Dose and directions for use, *see* ESERINE (111), PILOCARPINE (251), and INSTILLATION OF COLLYRIA (141).]

Contract the *pupil*.—*Lessen intraocular tension*.— Are *poisonous*.

Collyrium is kept aseptic and its action is not modified by adding 1 cc. of a 1 : 1000 sublimate solution to 10|0 of the collyrium.

To get the *greatest effect possible* the *pure salt* can be introduced, care being taken to compress lachrymal passages.

a. Eserine (physostigmine) (111). Active myotic, somewhat irritating to conjunctiva.

b. Pilocarpine (251). Less active but better tolerated by conjunctiva.—Particularly indicated in cases lasting some length of time.

c. Muscarine has been abandoned on account of its uncertain action.

236. NAPHTOL.

Naphtol *a* is more irritating than, but has twice the antiseptic strength of, naphtol *β*.

a. Naphtol *a*	0|20	3 gr.
Distilled water	1000|00	2 pts.

---

b Naphtol *a*	0|50	8 gr.
Lanolin	10|00	2½3

237. NEURALGIA OF THE FIFTH NERVE.

Laxatives.—Foot baths (118).—Galvanic current [positive electrode applied upon the painful part.]

Locally: Heat.—Massage and friction with: Spirits of camphor, soothing liniments (224), menthol pencil (228 *b*) or ointment (228 *a*), iodide of methyl (230).—Mustard plaster (288) or a vesicant applied at nape of the neck.

Internally: Antipyrin (15 *a*), antifebrin (14), gelsemium (121), phenacetin (248).

In *severe cases:* Hypodermic injection of morphine (231 *c*), of antipyrin (15 *b*), or of osmic acid (245).—Alternating hot and cold applications followed by energetic massage.—Neurectomy.

238. NEURITIS, OPTIC.—PAPILLITIS.—INTRABULBAR NEURITIS.—PAPILLARY STASIS.—NEURO-RETINITIS.—PERINEURITIS.

Treat the cause (meningitis, tumors, abscesses, etc.).—Combat circulatory troubles (dysmenorrhœa, etc.).

In *fresh cases:* Derivatives.—Dark room.—Pressure bandage.—Mydriatics (233).—Bloodletting (186) at the mastoid process.—Sweating (305).—Drastic cathartics.

Later: Dry leeches.—Preparations containing iodine (147 *b*).—Foot-baths (118).

In the *regressive stage:* Strengthening treatment.—Eye-douches (99).—Galvanic current.—Sojourn in the country.

Avoid: Sudden changes from a mild light into a bright light, congestions to the head, and excitement.

For those suffering from *rheumatism:* Alkalies (lithium (225), etc.); for *scrofulous* and *anæmic* patients: Iron (164), arsenic (20); for *syphilitic* patients: Specific treatment (291).

239. NEURITIS, RETRO-BULBAR.

Rest, light diet.—Energetic inunctions with mercury (143) *during three weeks; where cases then remain unimproved, cease.*—Bloodletting (186), foot-baths (118), derivative treatment.—Iodide of potassium (146 *b, c*), strychnine (300).—Diuretics, diaphoretics (305).

Nitrate of Silver. *See* SILVER (287).

240. OCCLUSIO PUPILLÆ.

Iridectomy or iridorrhexis.

Oil, Castor. *See* OLEUM RICINI (274).

Ointment, Blue = Simple Mercurial Ointment. *See* MERCURIAL INUNCTIONS (143).

Ointment, Calomel. *See* CALOMEL (33 *a, b*).

Ointment, Neapolitan = Double Mercurial Ointment. *See* SPECIFIC TREATMENT (291 *b*).

Ointment, Red. *See* MERCURY (229 *c*).

Ointment of Unna. *See* PEROXIDE OF HYDROGEN (135).

Ointment, Yellow. *See* MERCURY (229 *a, b*).

Ophthalmia of the New-Born. *See* BLENNORRHŒAL CONJUNCTIVITIS (69).

241. OPHTHALMIA, SYMPATHETIC.

Enucleation of the *eye first affected* and excision of part of the optic nerve, followed by an irrigation with a sublimate solution (1 to 2 per 1000) during five minutes.

Should the *eye first affected not be amaurotic* and the *other eye* already much diseased: *Symptomatic treatment:* Narcotics.—Atropine (23 *a*).—Dark room; absolute rest.—Iced compresses or hot poultices (255), according to the state in which the eye is.—Diuresis and diaphoresis (305).—Mercurial treatment (143, 291 b).

242. OPIUM.

a. Extract of opium . . . . 0|20   3 gr.
   Distilled water . . . . 100|00   3½ ℥
   Several instillations a day, 1 drop at each instillation.

b. Tincture of opium . . . . 10|0   2½ ℥
   10 to 20 drops at a time in brandy or upon a piece of sugar. A little water to be swallowed afterwards.

c. Extract of opium . . . . . . 0|02 to 0|06   ⅓ gr. to 1 gr.
   Subnitrate of bismuth . . } āā   0|5 āā 8 gr.
   Sugar of milk . . . . . }
   A powder; take two powders like this, the first one 1 1-2 hours, the second 1 hour before cataract operation.

243. OPTIC NERVE, ATROPHY OF THE.

Careful anamnesis and appropriate general treatment.

In the *beginning* of the atrophy: Injections of strychnine (300 a); iodide of potassium internally (146 c) and in inunctions (146 a, b).—Should there be *no improvement after several weeks:* Cease this form of treatment so as not to harm the general health, as the resulting benefit to vision is very problematical.

Preparations containing *iodine* (147 b) or *iron* (164).—*Hydrotherapy.* Douches in a stream along the spinal column.—Prolonged applications of heat or cold upon the vertebral column.—Sojourn in a warm climate.—Sweating (305).—*Massage* of the *eyeball.*—Galvanic current.

In case of *syphilis:* Specific treatment (291).

244. ORBICULAR MUSCLE, PARALYSIS OF THE.—LAGOPHTHALMUS.

Etiologic treatment. — Electricity. — Surgical treatment.—Compare also Keratitis through Lagophthalmus (168).

245. OSMIC ACID.

Osmic acid	0|05	1 gr.
Distilled water	10|00	$2\frac{1}{3}$

For hypodermic injections: One syringeful contains 0\|005 ($\frac{1}{10}$ gr.) osmic acid. Keep from light.

Ozæna. *See* RHINITIS (273).

Pagenstecher's Ointment. *See* MERCURY (229 *a, b*).

Pannus. *See* PANNOUS KERATITIS (172).

Panophthalmitis. *See* SUPPURATIVE CHOROIDITIS (48).

246. PARALYSIS AND PARESIS OF THE OCULAR MUSCLES.

Etiologic treatment.

In case of *rheumatism:* Large doses of salicylate of soda (275).—Sudorifics (305).

In case of *syphilis:* Energetic specific treatment (291).

Electricity: a. In paralysis of *peripheral origin:* *Galvanization.* The positive pole is a broad plate,

which is placed upon the neck or the arm. The negative pole has an ovoid form well adapted to the shape of the closed eye. A more circumscript effect is achieved by the use of lentiform electrodes. These should be well insulated with varnish and caoutchouc with the exception of one surface. The eye having been cocainized, the electrode is placed upon the globe directly as far as possible along the position of the diseased muscle. Duration of application one minute for each single muscle.—
b. In paralysis of *central origin: Faradization* of the brain may be tried. The electrodes are to be applied upon opposite sides of the head.

Should *diplopia trouble* the patient: *Prisms*, if the images are near enough to each other to be united by this means, which is *rarely* the case; *opaque glass,* where *distance* between images is too *great* to unite them.

Where above-named treatments give little or *no result: Surgical intervention.* Give patient binocular vision, at least in a part of the visual field, by a comprehensive advancement of the muscle combined with a tenotomy of its antagonist.

Paralysis of the Orbicular Muscle. *See* Orbicular Muscle (244).

247. PERMANGANATE OF POTASSIUM.

Permanganate of potassium . . 0|05 to 0|50 1 gr. to 8 gr.
Distilled water . . . .   200|00 6ʒ 4ʒ

This solution should not be used after it changes in color.

Peroxide of Hydrogen. *See* Hydrogen (135).

248. PHENACETIN.

Phenacetin . . . . } āā 0|50   8 gr.
Sugar of milk . . . .
From 1 to 3 powders a day in milk.

249. PHENOL.—CARBOLIC ACID.

a. Phenol . . . . 0|20   3 gr.
    White vaseline . . . . 10|00   2½ʒ

---

b. Phenol . . . . 4|0   1ʒ
    Distilled water . . . . 100|0   3℥ 2ʒ
    Instruments should remain in this solution for 45 minutes at least.

c. Phenosalyl. Mixture of carbolic acid, salicylic acid, lactic acid, menthol, and oil of eucalyptus. Takes the place of carbolic acid; is of greater antiseptic strength.
    It is used in the following proportions:

c'. 1 : 100 *for instruments.*
c''. 4 : 1000 *for the conjunctiva.*

Phlyctæna of the Conjunctiva and of the Cornea. *See* PHLYCTENULAR KERATITIS (173).

250. PHTHISIS OF THE EYEBALL.

Prothesis.—In case of persisting inflammatory symptoms: Enucleation.

As the phthisical eye is an organ which has kept its vitality, one must never forget telling patients that such an eye is a *permanent danger for the other eye* (ossification, cicatricial enclosure of the ciliary nerves, etc.)

Physostigmine. *See* ESERINE (111).

251. PILOCARPINE.

Hydrochlorate of pilocarpine	0|10	1½ gr.
Distilled water	10|00	2ʒ3

Instil 1 drop several times a day.

Pilocarpine *internally* and in *hypodermic* injections, see Methodical Sweating (305).

Poisoning by pilocarpine, see Methodical Sweating (305).

252. PINGUECULA.

The pinguecula may be left without any treatment, or can be removed for cosmetic purposes.

253. PLANTAIN.—AQUA PLANTAGINIS.

Soothing compresses; can be added to the different collyria.

Plaster of Mustard. *See* SINAPISM (288).

Poisoning by Atropine. *See* ATROPINE (23); **by Morphine**, *see* MORPHINE (231); **by Pilocarpine**, *see* METHODICAL SWEATING (305).

254. POTASSIUM ACETATE.

Acetate of potassium	4|0	1ʒ
Oxymel of squill	50|0	1ʒ 5ʒ
Distilled water	1000|0	2 pts.

Drink in one day; a wineglassful at a time.

255. POULTICES.

a. Potato starch poultices.

Dissolve starch in a quantity of water just sufficient to make a paste; upon this paste pour boiling water, stirring briskly, until the mixture is transparent and homogeneous. This mass is kept over the fire for 30 seconds, then wrapped in two squares of muslin which have been steeped in water previously in order to remove stiffness.—Heat the reserve poultice constantly in the water-bath while the other remains on the eye; change as soon as it begins to get cool.—Cover the poultice with a piece of flannel and a piece of oiled silk overlapping the poultice on all sides.

For antiseptic purposes boric acid (4 : 100) or sublimate (1 : 5000) can be used to dissolve the starch. Proceed in a *similar manner* for:

b. *Linseed* poultices.
c. *Bread* or *bread and bran* poultices.

Where *pains* are very *severe*:

d. Powdered hyoscyamus leaves . . . . 30|0 1ʒ
   Linseed-meal . . . . 100|0 3ʒ 2ʒ
   or:
e. Powdered conium leaves . . . . 40|0 1ʒ 2½ʒ
   Powdered belladonna leaves . . . . . . 20|0 5ʒ
   Water . . . . 1000|0 2 pts.
   Reduce one-fourth by boiling. Add linseed-meal q. s.

For *dry* poultices:

f. Aromatic leaves,
   or:
g. Conium leaves . . . . 50|0 1ʒ 5ʒ
   Species emollientes . . . . 150|0 5ʒ

256. PRESBYOPIA.

Where by presbyopia is understood an incapacity of prolonged eye-work, due to age on account of the diminution of the amplitude of accommodation, the *following table will show approximately the convex glass necessary to an emmetrope* for reading at a distance of *30 cm.*:

Years.	Diopters.
40	0.25
45	1.0
50	1.5
55	2.0
60	2.5
65	3.0
70	3.5

These numbers obtain for the emmetropic eye. The *hypermetrope* should *add* to the number corresponding to his age the lens correcting his hypermetropia, while the *myope* should *subtract* the glass correcting his myopia.

Work nearer by necessarily requires a stronger glass; farther off, a weaker one. Compare: Rules for prescribing glasses for work (125).

257. PTERYGIUM.

Ablation by any method permitting the bringing in contact of the margin of the cornea with healthy conjunctiva.—*Cauterize the corneal wound.*

258. PTOSIS.

Systemic treatment. — Electricity. — Surgical treatment.

259. QUININE.

a'. Wine of Calisaya bark.
 Small glassful with meals.

a''. Wine of Calisaya bark and iron	10|00	2⅓
Citric acid	2|50	40 gr.
Malaga wine	2000|00	4 pts.
Sugar	200|00	7ℨ

Tablespoonful 2 or 3 times a day.

b. Decoction of Calisaya bark . . . . 20\|0   5ℨ
    Water . . . . 200\|0   7ℨ
    Syrup of bitter orange peel . . . . . . 30\|0   1ℨ
    While boiling add:
Diluted sulphuric acid . . . . 0\|50   8 gr.
(In order to keep draught clear.)
    Tablespoonful 3 times a day.

c. Sulphate of quinine . . . . 0\|50   8 gr.
    A powder. Take one powder every 2 or every 4 hours.

Antipyretic.

260. RESORCIN.

a. Resorcin . . . . 1\|0   15 gr.
    Vaseline . . . . 10\|0   2⅓

    Resorcin spray:

b. Resorcin . . . . 5\|0   1⅓
    Distilled water . . . . 1000\|0   2 pts.

261. RETINA, ANÆMIA OF THE.

Systemic treatment [chlorosis, anæmia (164, 259), leucæmia, diseases of the heart].—Massage of the body and gymnastic exercises.—Hydrotherapy (98).

262. RETINA, ANÆSTHESIA OF THE.

Dark room; after the sixth day increase light gradually.—Later, smoked or blue glasses.—Absolute rest of the eyes for a long time.—Tonics.—

Bromides (31), lactate of zinc (325 d).—Hydrotherapy (98), salt and iron baths (25 c, d, e).—Inhalations of amyl nitrite (11).—Galvanic and faradic current.

Treat the cause [hysteria].—Suggestion.

263. RETINA, ASTHENOPIA OF THE.

Treatment for neurasthenia: Scottish douches (98 b), river baths, sojourn in the mountains or at sea-shore.

Stop sexual excesses (onanism) and excesses at table.—Smoked glasses.

Where photophobia is great, blow anæsthetic vapor into the external auditory canal.

264. RETINA.—"COMMOTIO RETINÆ."

Rest.—Dark room.—Cold compresses.

265. RETINA, DETACHMENT OF THE.

Dark room.—Atropine (23 a).—Remain in bed, lying upon the back, if possible (get up every other day for an hour or two, but during this time lie down on a lounge).—Avoid sudden movements.

Pressure bandage; change the bandage once or twice a day.

According to the general health of the patient: Every 5 days *bloodletting* (186) or dry leeches behind the ear.

Food that is easily digested, particularly milk. —No hard food requiring mastication.—Watch the stools.—*Derivative* and *diaphoretic* treatment (305).

Follow out this treatment for several weeks.—

Patient will slowly take up his habitual life, and should wear smoked or blue glasses for a long time.

Where there is no notable improvement: Try one of the following *operative procedures:*

Puncture or incision at the meridian of the sclera on a level with the detachment.—12 to 15 small *cauterizations* over the whole surface of the sclera corresponding to the detachment (avoid the ciliary zone); or *electrolysis:* A platin-iridium needle is attached to the positive pole. The negative electrode is placed upon the arm. The needle is introduced at the place of the detachment.—Current of 3 to 5 milliampères.—Duration of application: One minute.—Aseptic bandage.

In all of these methods of treatment a chance for improvement lies only in fresh cases and where the detachment is not too great in extent.

Prophylaxis: Individuals predisposed to a detachment of the retina, as myopes of a high degree, or those having already lost one eye through retinal detachment, should avoid sudden movements, congestions, constipation, strains, coughing, vomiting, overwork for the eyes, etc.

266. RETINA, HEMORRHAGES OF THE.

Systemic treatment [pernicious anaemia, diseases of the heart, nephritis], and treatment of the direct cause [congestions, indigestion, excitement, overwork, menstrual troubles].

Pressure bandage.—Absolute rest.—Cold compresses.—Bloodletting (186).—Foot-baths (118).—

Diuresis, cathartics, diaphoretics (305).—Iodide of potassium (146 c).

In *diabetes:* Strict diet: no sugar, no starch, saccharine, specially prepared bread.—Exercise of the body.—Arsenic (20).—Vichy water.

In case of frequent *relapses:* Ergot (109), to increase the tonus of the blood-vessels.

267. RETINA, HYPERÆMIA OF THE.

Treat the systemic trouble (anomalies of circulation, emphysema, etc.).—Rest the eyes [*no mydriatics* increasing hyperæmia of the fundus but rather myotics (235)].—Smoked glasses or dark room for some length of time.

Purgatives.—Bleeding (186) behind the ear.—Periodical and prolonged *cold applications* (compresses or ice-bag).

268. RETINA, HYPERÆSTHESIA OF THE.

Rest.—Dark room, later smoked glasses, the tint of which should be diminished gradually.—Where there is astigmatism correct it.

Systemic treatment for anæmia, chlorosis (164, 259), and the neuroses, which are often the cause of this affection.

269. RETINA, ISCHÆMIA OF THE.

Combat spasmodic interruption of the circulation by eye-douches (99) or alternate hot and cold compresses.—Absolute rest, dark room.—Digitalis (96), amyl nitrite (11).—Tonics, stimulants.

270. RETINA, TUMORS OF THE.

[Glioma, gliosarcoma, etc.]
Enucleation.

271. RETINITIS, DIFFUSE, Exudative, Punctated, Specific, Albuminuric, Diabetic, Leucæmic.

Treat the *systemic disease.*

In the *beginning:* Absolute rest in a dark room.—Henrteloup or leeches behind the ear (186), where general health of patient permits.—According to the constitution of patient: Iodide of potassium (146), mercury (229) or iron (164), quinine (259).—Mild purgatives.

Later: Smoked glasses; avoid sudden change from darkness to bright light.—Strengthening food, tonics, sojourn in the country or at the sea-shore.—In *unyielding cases:* Try repeated paracentesis.—*When cured:* Correct anomalies of refraction before permitting return to work.—Continue treatment, and long after re-establishment of vision take great care of the eyes.

272. RETINITIS PIGMENTOSA.—PIGMENTARY DEGENERATION OF THE RETINA.

No form of treatment is effective.—To retard development: Strengthening food.—Cod-liver oil (54).—Hydrotherapy (98).—Where the eyes are very sensitive to light: Dark glasses.

Retinitis, Purulent. See PURULENT CHOROIDITIS (48).

273. RHINITIS, CHRONIC.

Treat the *cause* [syphilis (291), scrofula, polyps].
Minute cleanliness.—Open air.—Good ventilation, particularly in the bedroom.

Spray the nose with a solution consisting of:

Peppermint water	100|0	3℥ 2½₰
Distilled water	200|0	6℥ 5₰
Glycerin	30|0	1℥
Biborate of soda	3|0	45 gr.

Nasal douches (100) with boric acid (4 : 100), permanganate of potassium (½ to 1 : 1000), or salt water (physiological solution 6 to 7 : 1000). In case of *ozæna* : Thymol (½ : 1000) or :

Salicylic acid	2|0	½₰
Biborate of soda	3|0	45 gr.
Distilled water	200|0	6℥ 4₰

Where there is *little secretion:* Prolonged inhalation of the steam of a saturated salt water solution. After each steaming use one of the following ointments :

White precipitate of mercury	0|50	8 gr.
Cold cream	25|00	6₰

or :

Sulphate of zinc	0|20	3 gr.
Vaseline	20|00	5₰

Every other day physician should apply :

Pure iodine	0|20	3 gr.
Iodide of potassium	0|30	5 gr.
Glycerin	30|00	1℥

to the nasal mucous membrane.

Where *secretion* is *copious* use one of the following powders as a snuff :

RICINI SALOL

Finely powdered betol .	. . . .	2|50	38 gr.
Menthol	. . . .	0|25	4 gr.
Pure cocaine	. . . . . .	0|10	1½ gr.
Ground roasted coffee	. . . . . .	1|50	23 gr.
Salicylate of bismuth	. . . .	15|00	1ʒ
Camphor		5|00	75 gr.
Pure cocaine		0|05	⅚ gr.

Atropic forms of ozæna require special treatment.

274. RICINI, OLEUM.—CASTOR OIL.

1 to 2 tablespoonfuls.
[Lemon juice may be added.]

275. SALICYLATE OF SODA.

Salicylate of soda.	6|0	1ʒ3
Distilled orange flower water . . . . . } āā 60|0		āā 2ʒ
Distilled peppermint water . . . . . . }		
Simple syrup	30|0	1ʒ

Tablespoonful every two hours.

276. SALICYLIC ACID.

Salicylic acid . . . . } āā 0|50 āā 8 gr.		
Tincture of benzoin . . . . }		
Lanolin	15|00	1ʒ

277. SALIPYRIN.

Combination of salicylic acid and antipyrin.—In powders of 0|5 (8 gr.).
From 1 to 4 powders a day.

278. SALOL.

Salol . . . . } āā 1|0		15 gr.
Sugar of milk . . . . }		

One powder; 4 to 10 powders a day.

Salt, Volatile = Carbonate of Ammonia.
See AMMONIA (10 *b*).

279. SCLERA, SUBCONJUNCTIVAL RUPTURE OF THE.

Absolute rest.—Pressure bandage.—Ice.

280. SCLERA, BENIGNANT TUMORS OF THE.

Expectant treatment.

281. SCLERA, MALIGNANT TUMORS OF THE.

Enucleation.

282. SCLERA, PENETRATING WOUNDS OF THE.

Suture the conjunctiva over the scleral wound.—Stitch at some distance from edge of wound so as to form a tampon of conjunctival tissue.

Where there is prolapse of the choroid coat: Replace it or cut it off (the latter measure is the safer).—Pressure bandage.—*Strict antisepsis.*—Absolute rest.

283. SCLERITIS.

Local treatment as in episcleritis (108), more or less energetic according to time of subsistence and intensity of inflammation.

Should this treatment not suffice: Leeches (186) at the temples.—Galvano-cautery or deep scarifications, followed by the instillation of a weak solution of eserine (111) or cocaine (52 *a*), and a dry bandage kept upon the eye night and day.—Galvanic current through a solution of salicylate of lithium [1 to 2 : 100], in which the eye is bathed for 5 minutes every other day.—During intervals: Dry heat or hot fomentations.—Foot-baths (118).

Treatment for *gout* and *rheumatism:* Salicylate of soda (275), antipyrin (15 *a*), antifebrin (14), tincture of aconite [*20 to 30 drops a day as a draught*], salicylate of lithium (225 *a*).

All *inflammatory symptoms* having *disappeared*, assist resorption by : Hydrotherapy (98).

Methodical sweating (305).—Compresses with :

Oil of turpentine	25|0	7ʒ
Yolk of one egg.		
Emulsify with a		
Chamomile infusion . . . . 15|0 to 300|0	½ʒ to 10ʒ	
Add		
Spirits of camphor	25|0	7ʒ
Shake the mixture before using.		

284. SCOPOLAMIN.

Hydrobromate (or hydrochlorate) of scopolamin	0|01 to 0|02	⅛ gr. to ⅓ gr.
Distilled water	10|00	2½ʒ
Instil 1 drop several times a day.		

Scotoma, Scintillant, with Objective Symptoms. *See* Synchisis (307).

285. SCOTOMA, SCINTILLANT, WITHOUT OBJECTIVE SYMPTOMS.

Tonics, good nourishment.—Avoid overwork.— *Stop* use of tobacco and of anything which can hinder digestion.—Antipyrin (15 *a*), quinine (259), caffeine [up to 1|0 a day].—Galvanic and faradic current.—Pressure on the suborbital nerves.—Repeated massage of the eyeball.—Suggestion.

Correct anomalies of refraction (particularly astigmatism) and of the accommodation.

Treat *hemicrania, anæmia, dyspepsia,* and other troubles, which generally accompany scintillant scotoma.

286. SECLUSIO PUPILLÆ.

Iridectomy.—Iridorrhexis.

287. SILVER, NITRATE OF.

a. Nitrate of silver . . . . 0|05   ⅝ gr.
   Distilled water . . . . 10|00   2½ ȝ

After instilling the collyrium neutralize with salt water. Keep solution from the light.

b. Nitrate of silver *pencil*.
   Pure nitrate of silver *pencil* (lunar caustic).
   Mitigated nitrate of silver *pencil*. Either:

a. Nitrate of silver . . . . } āā 1|5   āā 23 gr.
   Nitrate of potassium . . . . }

or:

β. Nitrate of silver . . . . 1|0   15 gr.
   Nitrate of potassium . . . . 2|0   ⅓ ȝ

After each application neutralize with salt water.

288. SINAPISM.

Dissolve mustard meal in barely lukewarm water and apply directly upon the skin.—Never use boiling water, vinegar, or acids.—Where *immediate effect* is desired use mustard paper.

Soothing Liniment. *See* LINIMENTS (224).

289. SPASM OF THE ORBICULAR MUSCLE, Tonic and Clonic.

Correct anomalies of refraction.—Treat existing conjunctivitis (70, 73, 78).

Smoked glasses, or dark room.—Leeches (186) at temple.—Injections of morphine (231 *c*).—Vapors inducing anæsthesia in the external auditory canal.—Keep from any irritation.—Bromides (31).—Tincture of aconite root [*20 to 30 drops daily as a draught.*]—Gelsemium (121).

In *persisting spasm:* Neurotomy or extirpation of the external nasal nerve.

290. SPECIES SUDORIFICÆ.

Adjuvant to diaphoretics and diuretics.

291. SPECIFIC TREATMENT. — ANTISYPHILITIC TREATMENT.

There are *three methods* of administering mercury, which should be applied according to the indication to be met.

a. Internal medication.—This is the *most practical* and the most simple method of administering mercury, *but* it naturally *depends upon* the *gastro-intestinal tolerance* of the patient.—It is not indicated in dyspepsia or any digestive troubles, tendency to diarrhœa, etc.—*a'*. Protiodide pills (5 centigr. for each pill with 1 centigr. of extract of opium). *1, later 2, of these pills a day just before meals.*—Or *a"*. Sublimate pills (302 *c*). *From 2 to 3 or even 4 of these pills a day where the stomach tolerates them. They should be taken immediately before or with meals.*

—Or *a'''*. Van Swieten's solution (302 *d*) (*1 or 2 tablespoonfuls a day in milk*).

b. *Method* of administering mercury *by inunctions.*—This method, while *very efficacious,* is often repellent to the patient on account of the *difficulties encountered in applying* it. Above all, there are dangers from irritation of the buccal cavity in it, which it is well to avert in time. The method is not indicated for patients with poor teeth or chronic gingivitis.—Daily inunctions (*lasting at least 10 minutes*) with 4|0 (1ʒ) of the double mercurial ointment (equal parts mercury and excipient). *These inunctions should be made alternately on one and on the other side of the body below the armpits.—Use ointment in the evening and leave it in contact with the skin over night.—Wipe off the ointment in the morning, wash with soap and powder with starch-meal.*

Watch the oral cavity during this treatment. Strict hygiene of the mouth.—Brush the teeth morning, night, and after meals.—Gargles of chlorate of potassium (*4|0 to one large glass of water*).—At the slightest trace of gingivitis suspend inunctions.

c. *Method* of administering mercury *by injections.* This is a *very active* method and in particular *acts quickly.* It is therefore to be preferred to the other methods where an imminent danger is to be averted or rapid action is indicated. However, it has its inconveniences, as it is *painful* and *produces* nodules or *sometimes* even *abscesses* at the seat of the injection.—It can be administered : (1) By daily injections of Delpech's solution (229 *n*) (*1 Pravaz syringeful*); or with the solution of the biniodide of

SPECIFIC TREATMENT

mercury in oil (229 i) *in the same dose:* or (2) the more active method with calomel injections at greater intervals can be employed:

Powdered calomel	1|0	15 gr.
Hydrocarbon oil	10|0	2⅓ ℥

*1 Pravaz syringe contains about 0|1 (1 1-2 gr.) of calomel.
—Dose: 1-2 Pravaz syringeful every week.*

Observe the usual rules of *strict antisepsis* while making these injections: Wash seat of injection previously with a sublimate or carbolic acid solution.—Use a syringe that can be sterilized; wash syringe with alcohol or carbolic acid solution; disinfect needle by heating.

Injection should *always* be a *deep* one. Deep injections are, as a rule, well borne by patients, while superficial injections are painful and dangerous at the same time.

These hypodermic injections can be made either in the retro-trochanteric fovea, the lumbar, or the gluteal region.

d. Combined treatment.

Where indications demand the *reënforcement of the action of mercury by that of iodide of potassium,* prescribe this drug and use in conjunction with mercurials:

d'. Distilled water	500|0	1 pt.
Iodide of potassium	30|0	1 ℥

2 to 4 tablespoonfuls before meals in 1-2 glass of milk, beer, or sugar water.

Or:

d''. Syrup of bitter orange peel	500|0	1 pt.
Iodide of potassium	25|0	6⅓ ℥

2 to 4 tablespoonfuls before meals in 1-2 glass of water.

One of the best methods of administering the combined treatment is the following: Immediately before each meal one (Dupuytren) sublimate pill (229 e) taken with a spoonful of the iodide solution or syrup.

Or: One injection or one daily inunction together with 2 to 3 to 4 tablespoonfuls of the iodide of potassium solution or syrup.

292. STAPHYLOMA, PARTIAL CORNEAL.

In a *recent* staphyloma: Repeated paracentesis followed by an aseptic pressure bandage.

Iridectomy.—Tattooing.—Excision of the cicatricial tissue.

Staphyloma, Pellucid Corneal. *See* KERATOCONUS (177).

293. STAPHYLOMA, TOTAL CORNEAL.

According to the degree of prominence: Tattooing or ablation with strict antiseptic precautions.

294. STAPHYLOMA, ANTERIOR SCLERAL.

Watch the case.—Where patient insists upon an operation: Ablation with strict antiseptic precautions.—Where staphyloma is very large and hinders the movements of the lids: Enucleation.

295. STRABISMUS, CONVERGENT NONPARALYTIC.

In *children under one year*: Do *not interfere.*— Later, atropine (23 a) (0|02 in 10|0 [$\frac{1}{3}$ gr. in $2\frac{1}{2}$5]); carefully instil one drop into each eye once or twice daily. For older patients use a stronger solution.—For children under three years give atropine in form of an ointment (23 d).—*Convex tinted glasses correcting* the *whole hypermetropia.*—Avoid looking near by as much as possible.—At an age where study is indispensable give for near vision convex glasses 3 D stronger than glasses used for distance, so as to be able to continue using mydriatic.

To develop *binocular vision:* Stereoscopic exercises repeated several times a day, even if only for a few minutes at a time.

This pacific treatment is continued as long as strabismus diminishes.—Should *strabismus* remain *stationary: Surgical intervention.* Where one eye has very poor vision, this should take place immediately. Where vision in both eyes is good: Operation can be postponed for months and years.

The surgical treatment which can be *most recommended* for convergent strabismus is the *advancement of the external recti of both eyes without tenotomy of the internal recti.* Advancement of the rectus externus of the strabotic eye alone will but *rarely* be sufficient.

After operation bandage both eyes and order patient to remain in bed until healing has taken place (6 days, as a rule).—When use of bandage is discontinued: Atropine, convex glasses, stereoscopic exercises until any tendency to strabismus has disappeared.

This treatment should *not* be *suddenly interrupted.* Begin by decreasing the dose of the mydriatic, later decrease strength of convex lenses. The glass correcting the manifest hypermetropia is retained as long as eye covered with the hand shows any tendency to convergence.—Watch and strengthen the general health.

Where strabismus is of *long standing*, of *high degree*, and where *motility* towards temples is *limited*, increase the effect of an advancement by *resection of the tendinous ends* of the external recti.—In the *highest degrees* only *tenotomy* of the internal rectus of the deviated eye may be *added*. But this tenotomy should be made *very cautiously* and not before several weeks or months have passed since the principal operation : *Horizontal* conjunctival incision, detachment of the tendinous end without lengthening the cut into Tenon's capsule.

In *over-correction:* Stop use of atropine, remove the binocular bandage as soon as possible, practise convergence.—Where necessary, reattachment of the retracted internal rectus by a suture.

In case of *insufficient correction :* At first energetic exercise without further surgical intervention.— Where insufficiency is due to the fact that the external rectus is attached too far away from the cornea, perform operation for the advancement of this muscle again.—It will hardly ever be necessary to perform tenotomy of both interni.

We would caution against the forced tenotomy as well as the "thread operation."—Prominence of the eyeball, retraction of the caruncula, restriction of the movement of the eye inward, and insufficiency of convergence may result, followed in most cases by a divergent strabismus.

296. STRABISMUS DEORSUM VERGENS.

If due to a *systemic disease:* Treat this disease. Should this not promise much : Surgical treatment.

Slight degree of strabismus deorsum vergens : Advancement of the superior rectus.

Medium degree: Extensive advancement of superior rectus with slight tenotomy of the inferior rectus.

High degree: Perform advancement of inferior rectus or tenotomy of superior rectus or both on the healthy eye in addition to the treatment mentioned above.

General rule: When a difference in the level of both eyes exists, it is better to place the eye which has the higher level on to a lower level (increasing the power of the inferior rectus by advancement), than to raise the other by a tenotomy of this muscle. As a matter of fact, the eyes are used more in lowering the glance than in looking up.

297. STRABISMUS, DIVERGENT NON-PARALYTIC.

Advancement of both internal recti will nearly always be necessary. Stereoscopic exercises greatly assist in this treatment.

In divergent strabismus of *long standing* and of *high degree* generally affecting an amblyopic eye, *tenotomy of the external rectus* must be *added* to a comprehensive advancement of the internus. Often even a combination of the advancement of both internal recti with a tenotomy of both external recti is necessary to achieve a sufficient correction. —Exercising convergence is useful to heighten the effect of the operation.

In *over-correction*: Reattach by advancement one of the muscles upon which tenotomy has been performed without touching those upon which advancement has already been practised.

Slight degrees of divergent strabismus are treated as Insufficiency of Convergence (142).

Strabismus, Paralytic. See PARALYSIS OF THE OCULAR MUSCLES (246).

298. STRABISMUS SURSUM VERGENS.

Where surgical treatment is indispensable:

Slight degree: Advancement of inferior rectus.

Medium degree: Advancement of inferior rectus with tenotomy of superior rectus, even detachment at its origin of the inferior oblique muscle.

Where the *degree* is *very high:* Assist these operations by a tenotomy of the inferior rectus of the other eye.

Compare also Strabismus Deorsum Vergens (296).

299. STROPHANTHIN.

Strophanthin . . . . 0|01 to 0|02 $\frac{1}{8}$ gr. to $\frac{1}{3}$ gr.
Distilled water . . . .   20|00 5$\bar{3}$

1 syringe = 0|0005 to 0|001 (1-125 gr. to 1-60 gr.) of strophanthin; injection 20 minutes before narcosis in case of disease of the heart.

300. STRYCHNINE.

a. Sulphate or nitrate of strychnine . . . . . 0|10   1$\frac{1}{2}$ gr.
Distilled water . . . .   10|00   2$\frac{1}{2}$$\bar{3}$

1 syringe = 0|01 strychnine; begin with 1-4 syringeful.

b. Sulphate or nitrate of strychnine . . . . 0|40   6 gr.
Lard . . . . 20|00   5ʒ
   Periocular inunctions, once or twice daily.

301. STYE. — HORDEOLUM. — FURUNCLE OF THE LIDS.

Poultices (255).—Incision followed by an antiseptic bandage (101).

As a prophylactic: Frequent sublimate washes (302 *b*); watch coexisting conjunctivitis (70) and blepharitis (26); derivative treatment.

302. SUBLIMATE, CORROSIVE = BICHLORIDE OF MERCURY.

a. Solution 1 : 500 : For disinfection of hands.— Treatment of purulent conjunctivitis and of granulations [friction of everted lids after massage with powdered boric acid].

b. Solution 1 : 5000 : The usual solution for washing and eye bandages.—For cataract operation add half the quantity of sterilized water.

These solutions [*a* and *b*] are *more efficacious* and will keep better *if* a quantity of chloride of sodium equal to that of sublimate is added.

c. Peptone . . . . 1|0   15 gr.
Distilled water . . . . 50|0   1ʒ 5ʒ
   Filter and add:
Corrosive sublimate solution 5 : 100 . . . . 20|0   5ʒ
Chloride of sodium solution 20 : 100 . . . . 16|0   ɫʒ
Distilled water, q. s. to make . . . . 100|0 3ʒ 2ʒ
   1 syringe = 0|01 (1-6 *gr*) *of sublimate.*

d. *Van Swieten's Solution:*

Corrosive sublimate	1|0	15 gr.
80 per cent. alcohol	100|0	3 ℥ 2ʒ
Distilled water	900|0	30 ℥

Not to be recommended *for local applications;* the alcohol contained in it is irritating to the eye.

e. *Dupuytren's Pills:*

Corrosive sublimate	0|50	8 gr.
Extract of opium	1|00	15 gr.
Extract of liquorice, q. s. for 50 pills.		

4 pills daily, to be taken immediately before or with meals.

Sublimate Baths. See MEDICATED BATHS (25).

303. SULFONAL.

2|0 to 4|0 *(1-2ʒ to 1ʒ) as a powder.—Before retiring.*

304. SULPHUR.

Precipitated sulphur	1|0	15 gr.
White vaseline	20|0	5ʒ

Application to remain on parts for several hours.

305. SWEATING, METHODICAL.—DIAPHORESIS.

In nearly all eye troubles *steam baths* are *contra-indicated*, as they cause congestion to the head. Only when every trace of inflammation is gone can they be used.

Sweating and salivation through pilocarpine:

a. As a draught [where stomach tolerates it]:

Hydrochlorate of pilocarpine	0|20	3 gr.
Brandy	20|00	5ʒ
Distilled water	250|00	8ʒ

2 to 4 tablespoonfuls daily, at intervals of 1-2 hour.

b. Hypodermic injections :

 Hydrochlorate of pilocarpine . . . . . . 0|10 1½ gr.
 Distilled water . . . . 10|00 2⅔ℨ

 Dissolve and filter; 1 syringe = 0|01 (1·6 gr.) of pilocarpine; 1 to 2 syringefuls a day.

To *assist sweating* and as a *diuretic* prescribe : Tea of species sudorificæ (290), of linden flowers, of sambucus, of quassia or the acetate of potassium (254).

In case of *pilocarpine poisoning :*

α. Absorption by gastro-intestinal tract :
 Stomach-pump or hypodermic injections of a solution of hydrochlorate of apomorphine (*2 : 100*), *up to 0 | 03 (1-2 gr.).*

β. Absorption through the tissues (injections) :
 Hypodermic injection of one milligramme of neutral sulphate of atropine [*2-10 of a Pravaz syringeful of the ordinary collyrium (23 a)*].

In both cases internally : Black coffee, brandy, carbonate of ammonia (10 *b*).

306. SYMBLEPHARON.

Surgical treatment.

307. SYNCHISIS, SCINTILLANT.—SCINTILLANT SCOTOMA, WITH OBJECTIVE SYMPTOMS.

[Crystals of cholesterin and tyrosine in the vitreous.]

Combat biliary lithiasis depending on alcoholism or arthritis.—Repeated paracentesis where there is also cholesterin or tyrosine in the aqueous humor.

Syphilis. *See* SPECIFIC TREATMENT (291).

308. SYRUPUS ARMORACIÆ.

Simple or with iodine.
A small glassful at meals.

309. TALC.

Dust upon integuments [moist and excoriated parts].

310. TANNIN.—TANNIC ACID.

a. Pure tannin . . . . 0|25   4 gr.
 Fennel water . . . . 20|00   5ʒ
 Distilled water . . . . 100|00   3℥ 2ʒ

b. Tannin . . . . } āā 10|0 āā 2½ʒ
 Glycerin . . . .   }
 Glycerole of starch . . . . 50|0   1℥ 5ʒ
 Apply to excoriated parts.

311. TARSITIS.

Antisyphilitic (291) or antiscrofulous treatment [iron (164), arsenic (20), cod-liver oil (54)].

Massage on a plate lid holder with an anodyne ointment or simple mercurial ointment. — Hot fomentations.—Scarifications.

312. THYMOL = THYMIC ACID.

Can replace phenol; as a spray (½ to 1 : 1000) upon the closed lids.

To make a 1 : 1000 solution : Dissolve the thymol in 4|0 (1ʒ) of 90 per cent. alcohol before adding water.

313. TILIÆ, AQUA.

Soothing compresses.—Can also be added to the different collyria.

Trachoma. *See* GRANULAR CONJUNCTIVITIS (75).

314. TRICHIASIS.

Destroy root of lashes by electrolysis. [*See* DISTICHIASIS (97).]

315. TRIONAL.

1|0 to 1|50 (15 gr. to 23 gr.) in a cup of hot milk before retiring.

316. TRYPSIN.

10 : 100 solution; dissolves diphtheritic membranes.

Tylosis. *See* LIDS (219).

Ulcer, Indolent. *See* NEUROPARALYTIC KERATITIS (171).

Ulcer of the Cornea. *See* ULCEROUS KERATITIS (176).

Unna's Ointment. *See* PEROXIDE OF HYDROGEN (135).

317. VASELINE.

Good excipient for eye salves; does not irritate; does not change when exposed to air.—In summer add a little ceresin or simple wax to keep it from getting too liquid.

White vaseline is the best as long as it is pure; when not sure of its quality take the yellow by preference.—Vaseline must be tasteless, odorless, and neutral.

318. VERATRINE.

Veratrine	0|50	7½ gr.
Lard	20|00	5ʒ

Periocular inunctions; once or twice daily.

319. VITREOUS, CYSTICERCUS OF THE.

Sufficiently long incision [not less than 8 mm.] in the direction of the cysticercus, following as much as possible a meridian of the eyeball.—Extraction with a hook, forceps, or by aspiration.—Sutures, antiseptic bandage (101).

Possibility of the presence of a second cysticercus!

320. VITREOUS, DETACHMENT OF THE.

Absolute rest.—Atropine (23 a).—Pressure bandage.—Diaphoresis (305), diuresis, laxatives.—*See* DETACHMENT OF THE RETINA (265).

321. VITREOUS, FOREIGN BODY OF THE.

Extraction with the electro-magnet, or, according to the case, with a hook or the forceps. Incision of the sclera in the region of the foreign body; sutures; antiseptic bandage (101).—This operation can be performed even when suppuration has begun around a piece of metal.—In case of *extensive suppuration: Enucleation or evisceration.*

322. VITREOUS, HEMORRHAGES INTO THE.

Treat the systemic disease: Nephritis, diabetes, pernicious anæmia.—Special treatment of the choroiditis (47) and chorio-retinitis (271).

Hemorrhage from *circulatory troubles* or *trauma:* Absolute rest, darkened room.—Atropine (23 *a*).—Pressure bandage.—Cupping at the temple.—Iced compresses upon the eye.

Later diaphoresis, diuresis, laxatives [pilocarpine (305), salicylate of soda (275), calomel (33 *d*)]. —Iodide of potassium (146 *c*).—Hot compresses.— Local douches alternately hot and cold.—Repeated paracentesis.

323. VITREOUS, LIQUEFACTION OF THE.—SYNCHISIS.

Treat the systemic disease.—*See* CHOROIDITIS (47) and RETINITIS (271).

324. VITREOUS, OPACITIES OF THE.

Special treatment of the choroiditis (47) and retinitis (271).

Derivative treatment, pilocarpine (305), iodide of potassium (146 *c*).—Galvanic current.—Prolonged poultices (255) upon the eye.—Where *thick central membranes* are found a discission should be made and the membranes can be displaced. [Scleronyxis.]

White Precipitate. *See* MERCURY (229).

Xerosis. *See* CONJUNCTIVA (67).

325. ZINC.

a. Sulphate or sulphophenate of zinc . . . . }	0|10 to	0|20	1½ gr. to 3 gr.
Distilled rose water . . .		50|00	1⅗ ʒ
Distilled water		150|00	5 ʒ
Mix and filter.			

ZONA OPHTHALMICA

b. Oxide of zinc . . . .   0|50 7½ gr.
   Vaseline . . . . 15|0 to 25|00 ʒ̃ to 6ʒ̃

c. Chloride of zinc . . . .   0|20   3 gr.
   Distilled water . . . .   30|00   1ʒ̃
   Tincture of opium . . . . 10 drops. 10 gtt.
   Filter.

d. Lactate of zinc . . . . 0|30   4½ gr.
   1 powder every 3 hours.

326. ZONA OPHTHALMICA.

Cupping (60|0 to 80|0 [2ʒ̃ to 2ʒ̃ 5ʒ̃]) near orifice of external nasal nerve.—Atropine (23 a).—Antiseptic bandage (101).—Washes and hot compresses, with:

Neutral acetate of lead . . . . 3|0   45 gr.
Powdered alum . . . . 2|0   ½ʒ̃
Distilled sterilized water. . . . . 150|0   5ʒ̃

For *pain:* Instillations of cocaine (52 a), injections of morphine (231 c) at the temple.

Internally: Quinine (259), antipyrin (15 a), antifebrin (14), or:

Fluid extract of gelsemium . . . . 1|0   15 gr.
Sulphophenate of sodium . . . . 7|0   1½ʒ̃
Distilled water . . . . 150|0   5ʒ̃
   Mix; teaspoonful every 2 hours.

Where vesicles having burst become *ulcers:*

Apply antiseptic washes (sublimate 1:2000), boric acid 4:100, etc., and later on ointments with calomel (33 *a, b*) or yellow oxide of mercury (229 *a, b*).

THE END.

Therapeutics:
ITS PRINCIPLES AND PRACTICE.

A work on Medical Agencies, Drugs, and Poisons, with Especial Reference to Relations between Physiology and Clinical Medicine.

By H. C. WOOD, M.D., LL.D.,

Professor of Materia Medica and Therapeutics, and Clinical Professor of Diseases of the Nervous System in the University of Pennsylvania

---

NEW TENTH EDITION.

Thoroughly Revised. 1 vol. Octavo. Over 1000 pages.

Cloth, $6.00; Sheep, $6.50.

NOTICE OF NINTH EDITION.

"To review this standard work is a real pleasure: it discovers so much original investigation, sound learning, and practical worth, and so little subservience to mere authority, that it engages attention, commands respect, and inspires confidence,—the chief *desiderata* in all teaching. Eliminating the effete material of former editions, discussing the newer remedies,—both official and non-official, and noting the latest advances in one of the most important branches of medicine, the author keeps his 'Therapeutics' as it has been nearly two decades,—abreast of the times, in the front rank of its kind, and nowise lacking. Especial attention is given the physiological action of drugs, without a fair knowledge of which, in our opinion, their clinical use is, as a rule, irrational, unsatisfactory, and, consequently, injurious; and the whole subject-matter evidences an intimate acquaintance with the topics considered, a keen conception of professional needs, and a judicious determination of authorial effort. Rarely, indeed, are the conservatism of the past and the enterprise of the present so happily blended,—a reasonable indication, perhaps, of its continued usefulness and popularity."—*Massachusetts Medical Journal.*

J. B. LIPPINCOTT COMPANY, Publishers,
PHILADELPHIA.

The Practice of Medicine.

By HORATIO C. WOOD, M.D., LL.D. (Yale),

Professor of Therapeutics and Clinical Professor of Nervous Diseases in the University of Pennsylvania; Member of the National Academy of Science,

AND

REGINALD H. FITZ, A.M., M.D.,

Hersey Professor of the Theory and Practice of Physic in Harvard University; Visiting Physician to the Massachusetts General Hospital; formerly Shattuck Professor of Pathological Anatomy in Harvard University.

Complete in one handsome octavo volume of about one thousand one hundred pages.

Cloth, $6.00; Sheep, $7.00; Half Russia, $7.50.
Sold only by subscription.

"The work before us is a good one in every respect, and is in addition a splendid example of collaboration in writing."—*St. Louis Medical and Surgical Journal.*

"It is a delight to pick up a work devoted to the practice of medicine which, instead of being a mere collation, is wholly original. This is but the second book of this precise character—the first by the same publishers—that has appeared in more than a quarter of a century."—*Detroit Medical Age.*

"Its information is sound, and is conveyed in a practical way."—*British Medical Journal.*

"A rather careful perusal of this book has convinced the reviewer that it is trustworthy, well-balanced, judicious, and modern. It is not padded; it is complete."—*Annals of Surgery.*

"This work is a departure from ordinary books upon the practice of medicine. It attempts, as the preface states, to treat the subject from the pathologic and therapeutic standpoint. The articles are signally brief, yet they go right to the centre of the topics and leave off the superfluous in a marked manner."—*Medical Journal*, Charlotte, N. C.

J. B. LIPPINCOTT COMPANY, Publishers,
PHILADELPHIA.

System of Diseases of the Eye.

BY AMERICAN, BRITISH, DUTCH, FRENCH, GERMAN, AND SPANISH AUTHORS.

EDITED BY

WILLIAM F. NORRIS, A.M., M.D.,

AND

CHARLES A. OLIVER, A.M., M.D.

Illustrated with engravings throughout the text, and numerous plates in both black and white colors. To be complete in four handsome imperial octavo volumes of about 600 pages each. Published at intervals of a few months. Octavo.

Cloth, $5.00; Sheep, $6.00; Half Leather, $6.50. Volume I. and Volume II. ready. Volume III. In preparation. For sale by subscription only.

"If the first volume of the 'System of Diseases of the Eye' reflects the greatest credit upon those who have compiled it, the publishers are entitled to at least equal praise. The general get-up, the paper, the type, the plates (including the figures interspersed in the text) have not been equalled in any work on ophthalmology. At the end of the book, which is tastefully bound, will be found a list of fifty-four contributors and the contents of the three volumes which are still to appear."—E. LANDOLT, in *Archives d'Ophthalmology*.

J. B. LIPPINCOTT COMPANY, Publishers,
PHILADELPHIA.

www.ingramcontent.com/pod-product-compliance
Lightning Source LLC
Chambersburg PA
CBHW030358170426
43202CB00010B/1411